FUELLING THE CYCLING REVOLUTION

FUELLING THE CYCLING REVOLUTION

The Nutritional Strategies and Recipes Behind Grand Tour Wins and Olympic Gold Medals

Nigel Mitchell

BLOOMSBURY
LONDON · OXFORD · NEW YORK · NEW DELHI · SYDNEY

Bloomsbury Sport

An imprint of Bloomsbury Publishing Plc

50 Bedford Square	1385 Broadway
London	New York
WC1B 3DP	NY 10018
UK	USA

www.bloomsbury.com

BLOOMSBURY and the Diana logo are trademarks of Bloomsbury Publishing Plc

First published in 2017

Text © Nigel Mitchell, 2017

Food photography by Adrian Lawrence
© Bloomsbury Publishing, 2017
Food styling by Emily Kydd

British Library Cataloguing-in-Publication Data

A catalogue record for this book is available from the British Library.

ISBN: Paperback: 9781472936936

ePub: 9781472936943

ePDF: 9781472936912

1 2 3 4 5 6 7 8 9 10

Designed in Futura, Lobster 1.4 and Wicked Grit by Saffron Stocker

Printed and bound in China by Toppan Leefung Printing

Bloomsbury Publishing Plc makes every effort to ensure that the papers used in the manufacture of our books are natural, recyclable products made from wood grown in well-managed forests. Our manufacturing processes conform to the environmental regulations of the country of origin.

To find out more about our authors and books visit www.bloomsbury.com. Here you will find extracts, author interviews, details of forthcoming events and the option to sign up for our newsletters.

CONTENTS

Introduction 6

1 THE NUTS AND BOLTS OF NUTRITION 11

2 GUT HEALTH: WORKING FROM THE INSIDE OUT....................... 25

3 OPTIMAL HYDRATION............ 41

4 THE DAY BEFORE 59

5 BREAKFAST....................... 75

6 EATING ON THE BIKE 93

7 RECOVERY.....................119

8 WEIGHT MANAGEMENT 141

9 SUPPLEMENTS 163

10 SPECIAL DIETS AND NUTRITIONAL NEEDS 189

11 NUTRITIONAL TIMELINES 213

Appendix 1: Urine Colour Chart.........228

Appendix 2: Carbohydrate Exchange List Ready Reckoner 229

Appendix 3: Ready Reckoner of Protein Foods 233

Appendix 4: Conversion Chart for Common Measurements 235

Acknowledgements 236

Index 237

INTRODUCTION

In the UK, with the Great Britain Cycling Team dominating at the Olympics and major championships and Team Sky winning the Tour de France with both Sir Bradley Wiggins and Chris Froome, cycling has undergone a revolution. With membership of British Cycling swelling, numerous sportives selling out within minutes of going live and more riders joining their local Sunday club run, cycling is no longer a minority sport.

Whether you're an aspiring racer looking to move up through the categories, training for a sportive or charity ride, or just wanting to be able to ride that bit faster, nutrition is key. Too many riders focus solely on tangible and visible external factors, such as the latest must-do training sessions or second-shaving aerodynamic or lightweight kit. They miss out the fundamental of the fuel they provide for their engine. You wouldn't expect a car to run on the wrong type of fuel, so why would you expect your body to perform on the wrong type of fuel either?

On or off the bike, the food you eat, when you eat it and in what quantities will have a profound effect on both your health and cycling performance. It's not just about preventing the 'bonk' on a long ride, but using diet and nutrition to enhance your recovery, adaptation to training and make you a better cyclist.

No sport from a nutritional perspective is totally unique. Cycling has some unique demands and qualities. The first is the sheer amount of work done in both racing and training. No other sport has races that are three weeks long, and even amateur riders think nothing of a four- to six-hour weekend ride backed up with three or four other sessions during the week. This puts massive physiological demands on the body. These demands cause the body to adapt and become fitter and stronger, but they can also cause it to start breaking down. Optimal nutrition supports the positive effects of training and helps to counter the negative. The second unique aspect is that you can eat and drink while riding. You certainly can't do this playing football and even distance runners don't have the same nutritional freedom and choices as cyclists. Knowing how to take advantage of this is essential for cycling performance and, if you fail to master this aspect of the sport, you'll never reach your potential.

My life in nutrition

My earliest sports nutrition memory is standing by the side of the road and handing my mother rice pudding to eat as she took part in a 12-hour time trial. This was her fuel of choice en route to logging an impressive 218 miles and it always makes me chuckle that both Sir Bradley Wiggins and Chris Froome's Tour de France wins were also rice-fuelled, in the form of my rice cakes, proving that not all nutrition is cutting-edge science. I loved supporting my mother in her races, but my mother's prowess in the kitchen wasn't nearly so impressive as her riding (spam fritters being her speciality), so this also fired up my interest in food and nutrition. I began talking to other local riders and making suggestions as to what they could try to improve their riding, whether it was a bigger breakfast or eating scones with jam on the bike – simple stuff, but all about getting some fuel into them.

When I left school, there was no real pathway into sports nutrition, so I decided to train as a clinical dietician. It's important to make a distinction between a dietician and a nutritionist. To be a dietician, you have to attain a recognised clinical qualification. This qualifies you to use nutrition in a clinical setting as a therapeutic tool and it's a protected title. Anyone can call themselves a nutritionist, regardless of qualifications, so you should always be wary who you take advice from. All the time while studying for my dietetics degree, I was thinking how I could apply what I was learning to sport. On graduating, I went to work in the NHS which was where I gleaned some of the most valuable knowledge that I'm now able to utilise with top athletes. It led me into situations where I was challenging the accepted dogma and looking for new solutions to problems. An example was weight management, working with patients suffering with cancer, diabetes and HIV/AIDS. The emphasis had always been on simple calories and energy balance, but I saw that, for preserving lean tissue mass, the key was protein. I also looked at the therapeutic benefit of essential fats, such as fish oils.

After the woeful performance of the Great Britain team at the 1996 Atlanta Olympics, there was a massive injection of public money into sports. More universities were offering sports science degrees and I became a lecturer in sports nutrition at Sheffield Hallam University in the UK. This allowed me to teach, conduct research and develop a consultancy. I was able to explore how what I'd learned in the clinical world could be applied to elite-level competition, and I began working across a whole range of sports including boxing, swimming and of course cycling.

I began working for British Cycling in 2002. British Cycling really embraced a progressive attitude regarding how athletes should be prepared for competition and left no stone unturned looking for those performance edges. The tales of the Secret Squirrel Club constantly tinkering with kit and trying new things are now legendary and we were doing the same with nutrition too. I remember working with Wiggins, who was riding the Giro d'Italia for his pro team and we put together a support package to get him through this three-week Grand Tour healthily. This included upping his protein and essential fat intake, and it worked.

Doping was still rife in professional cycling. The accepted wisdom was that you couldn't get through a Grand Tour without some form of artificial assistance. This may not have been by illegal doping, but dubious practices were all seen as mandatory. We refused to accept this and our message was that you could be the best without drugs.

The next step was a professional road team and, in 2009, this happened with Team Sky. Pro cycling was an incredibly traditional sport that was set in its ways, but we really shook things up. Other teams and the media ripped into us about getting our riders to cool down on turbos after a hard mountain-top finish, but now you see virtually every team doing it. It was the same with my nutritional approach. The emphasis in cycling had always been on the importance of carbohydrates and, it's true, you can't ride well without them. However, I saw that you had to periodise your eating based on the training and racing you're doing. If you overeat carbs, you get fat. If you don't eat enough, you can't ride hard. It's about finding the balance and eating appropriately.

There are plenty of lessons to learn from the past – my mother's liking for rice pudding on the bike being one. Wiggins mentioned that he'd loved rice cakes, so I reworked a recipe for him, and now almost every pro team has their own version. I also remember talking to former professional rider Max Sciandri, who complained about always having a swollen belly in the final week of a Grand Tour, which led me to really look into ways to maintain gut health and function. After all, there's no point taking on nutrients if you can't digest and absorb them. I was lucky enough to work with Sean Yates and he told me that one of his weight-loss strategies had been big rides on a spoonful of olive oil. It needed tweaking and refining, but the idea was basically the same as the low carbohydrate training we do today.

After 12 years with British Cycling and six with Team Sky, it was time for me to move on. The structure and resources at Cannondale are completely different and it's given me the scope to completely rewrite their nutritional rulebook and protocols. I'm working with their nutritional supplier and am also really able to explore the nutritional implications of power meter data, potentially a really exciting area.

By taking the time to read and understand this book, you'll benefit from my 25 years of clinical and sports experience. You'll better understand your body, the food you put into it and the impact good nutrition can have. Nutrition may not be as exciting or instantly gratifying as a flash new set of deep section wheels, but I can guarantee, if you follow my advice, it'll have a far greater impact on your cycling performance.

Nigel Mitchell

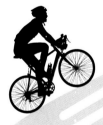

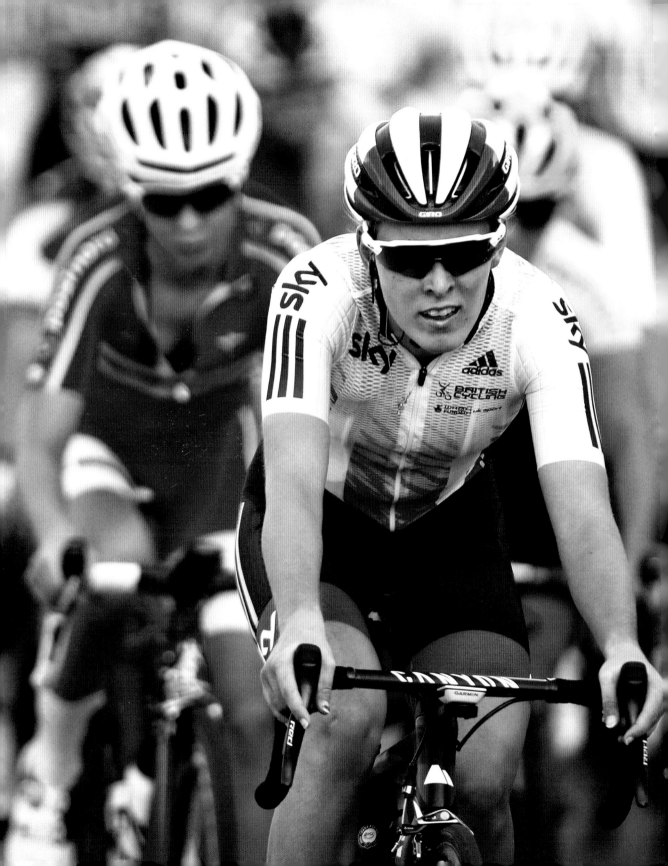

THE NUTS AND BOLTS OF NUTRITION

Eating is a necessity of life. We go through the daily routine of breakfast, lunch and dinner, often with little thought or consideration to what we're actually putting into our mouths: just grabbing a sandwich and eating it at our desks, hurriedly eating a slice of toast as we rush for the train or mindlessly consuming dinner in front of the TV once the kids are finally in bed. Evolution has thankfully programmed us to seek and crave the basic nutrients to survive but, if you're interested in optimum performance and health, a more informed, mindful and disciplined approach is necessary. Equate your diet to building a bike and I know you wouldn't do that without a lot of thought and research. The basics are the frame, but even these can range from basic alloy (think supermarket budget) to top-of-the-range carbon fibre, ethically produced and sourced organic. You've then got your wheels and components to consider, and, with this book, I'll give you the tools to finish your build with Dura-Ace rather than Claris.

MACRONUTRIENTS: THE 'GO NUTRIENTS'

The macronutrients are carbohydrates, proteins and fats. These provide the body with energy and its basic building blocks. They are essential to function and I consider these to be the nutrients that make you 'go'.

The sun is the source of all our energy. Plants use the energy from sunlight to make carbohydrate through photosynthesis. Animals then eat the plants and, in turn, use or store the carbohydrates as energy. When we eat the animals and plants, we absorb these carbohydrates and their energy is released through respiration. It's an energy chain. When I teach athletes about nutrition, I use this simple process to explain where this energy comes from so they can appreciate the steps which are needed for us to function, train and race.

Carbohydrates

Carbohydrates used to be the main focus of endurance sports nutrition. Who can forget the pasta parties that were seen as mandatory the evening before a big marathon? Carbohydrates are the body's main source of energy, especially when working hard, but we now know that more isn't necessarily more and that their consumption has to be balanced and controlled.

Carbohydrates exist in the form of sugars and starches. All carbohydrates are simply one or many glucose molecules linked together. Table sugar, or sucrose, is composed of two sugar molecules (a glucose and fructose), whereas a complex carbohydrate, such as maltodextrin, is a chain of many. Once in the body, all carbohydrates are broken down into glucose for immediate use or converted into a starch known as glycogen, which is stored in the liver and muscles for later use. These stores are fairly limited and only have energy to fuel about 90 minutes of exercise. Once these stores are full, excess carbohydrates are converted to, and stored as, fat.

The carbohydrates that you take on during a ride, by sipping on a sports drink, using a gel or eating a slice of cake at the rest stop, supplement the energy available from your glycogen stores and mean you can keep on riding for far longer than 90 minutes. How quickly that energy is available is determined by the complexity (the number of linked glucose molecules) of the carbohydrates you consume. More complex carbohydrates will yield their energy more gradually whereas simple carbohydrates (sugars) will give an almost instantaneous hit. You need a combination of simple and complex carbohydrates on the bike and, if you look at the ingredients in many gels and sports drinks, you'll see this need addressed. Remember, the harder you're working, the higher the proportion of carbohydrates you'll use.

Off the bike, carbohydrates are important, but their consumption has to be in proportion to the training and intensity of workouts you're performing. Just because you're a cyclist doesn't mean you need to continuously eat vast mountains of pasta. Even when fuelling riders on Grand Tours the carbohydrate heavy emphasis has definitely shifted. However, some nutritionists and riders take this too far and are compromising training and racing performance by not allowing enough carbohydrates. It's all about the correct amounts at the right time and we'll discuss this fully in later chapters.

Not all carbohydrates found in food are digestible and usable as energy by humans. Plant cellulose is a non-digestible starch found in fruit and vegetables. This fibre, though, plays a vital role in maintaining gut health and is an essential component in a healthy and balanced diet. There are two main types of fibre, soluble and insoluble. Insoluble fibre helps to form the bulk of the stool and soluble fibre acts as a lubricant to keep the stool soft. Foods such as oats are great sources of soluble fibre whereas wholemeal bread is insoluble.

Proteins

Proteins are composed of molecules known as amino acids and these can truly be thought of as the building blocks of life. All of the proteins in our bodies are arrangements of the 20 amino acids and all proteins we consume are broken down in the gut into their constituent amino acids. Eight of these amino acids are described as essential. This is because they cannot be synthesised in our bodies and therefore must be consumed in our diet. Animal protein sources contain all of the essential amino acids and are referred to as 'complete proteins', however, many plant proteins are not complete. It's therefore vital for vegans and vegetarians to consume a wide variety of plant proteins to ensure they obtain all the essential amino acids.

Once consumed and broken down into amino acids, protein is used by the body for the production of its own proteins, such as

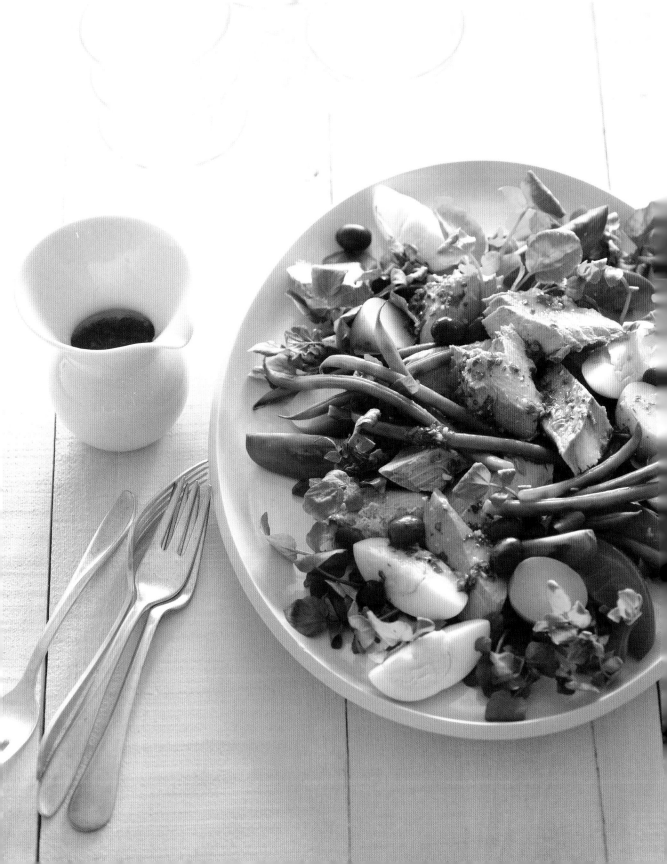

muscle, in its primary function of growth and repair. This is why taking on some protein is so important after a long and hard ride. It's responsible for repairing all the microtraumas you've caused to your muscles and, in doing so, allows the muscles to adapt to the training and become stronger. Proteins are also used in making essential hormones, enzymes and supporting immune function. In certain situations, usually when all other fuels have been exhausted, proteins can also be broken down and used as an energy source. If you fail to fuel your body sufficiently, especially if inflicting a crash diet on yourself, your body will actually sacrifice and break down its own protein, your muscles, to provide fuel.

The importance of protein in strength and powerbased sports has long been recognised, but it's only more recently that its necessity for endurance athletes has been discovered. We now know that adequate quality protein is one of the key nutritional requirements for a rider completing a Grand Tour healthily and to the best of their ability. For amateur riders too, the optimal amount of protein is essential and, if you've typically followed a more carbohydrate-heavy traditional cycling diet, you may find the switch of emphasis to protein takes a little getting used to.

Even on the bike, we've experimented and had success with riders consuming protein. Carbohydrate-fasted rides, where riders head out without breakfast or have a protein-only breakfast such as an omelette, have been used for a long time by riders looking to get lean and improve their fat-burning ability. However, more recently on these type of rides, we've been giving riders protein drinks and have found that it enhances both their adaptation and recovery. When he was losing weight and transforming himself from a track cyclist to a Grand Tour winner, Sir Bradley Wiggins would do six-hour steady-paced rides using protein alone at Team Sky's Majorcan training camps.

Fats

Fats were once considered to be totally off limits to serious cyclists, with a low-fat and high-carbohydrate diet the norm for all endurance athletes. However, like protein, we now know that the right types of fat in the correct amounts are as important to performance and well-being as carbohydrates and don't result in uncontrollable weight gain.

Stored fat is the body's go-to energy source during steady state exercise. It's a bit like the body's diesel, excellent for long and slow, with carbohydrates being the higher octane fuel for more intense activities. The more adapted you are to an activity the better you'll be able to tap your fat reserves and, with even a super-lean cyclist carrying about 100,000 kcal worth of energy in fat, being able to use it certainly makes sense. If you're able to burn fat efficiently, you'll spare your limited glycogen supplies and won't have to walk on such a nutritional knife-edge and won't be totally reliant on topping up your carbohydrate reserves as you ride. This is essentially the physiological ability that Sean Yates was training with on his epic, olive oil-fuelled rides.

Along with providing an energy source, fats supply the body with essential fatty acids that it cannot synthesise. These include omega-3 fatty acids, found in fish oils and flaxseeds, which we've found to be extremely beneficial to cyclists. Fats are important for the absorption of fat-soluble vitamins and also provide foods with flavour and texture.

There are three main forms of dietary fat: saturated, unsaturated and trans fats. Saturated fats are typically found in animal sources, such as meat and dairy, whereas unsaturated fats tend to come from plants. The terms 'saturated' and 'unsaturated' simply refer to the structure of the fatty acids that comprise the fat, in particular the bonds that hold their structure together. Unsaturated fats have 'double' bonds and tend to be liquid at room temperature. Rich sources of unsaturated fats include olive oil, avocados, nuts and fish. Saturated fats have no double bonds and are solid at room temperature. Fat structure is important because these double bonds and the sequence they appear in affects how the body uses them and their function.

Trans fats are found in commercially produced baked goods, snacks and some margarine. These are produced by using hydrogen to change the structure of an unsaturated fat so it is easier to use in food production. Generally, you should be looking to replace saturated and trans fats with more unsaturated fats.

Alcohol

Alcohol is a fourth, but non-essential and unfortunately not very effective, energy source for the body. The attitude to alcohol has changed significantly in pro cycling. At one time, drinks such as brandy were given to help fortify riders on the bike and often riders would stop for a beer on hot days. Today, alcohol is generally avoided by serious riders during racing and training blocks. One gram of alcohol will provide approximately 7 kcals of energy, but, unfortunately, from an exercise point of view, the energy from alcohol is practically worthless. The alcohol is generally converted to fat in the liver then circulated around the body. Alcohol can act as a diuretic (i.e. cause you to lose more fluid then consumed), can also slow healing from injury, and affect your recovery from workouts. During racing pro riders tend to steer clear of alcohol, with the exception of a glass of champagne if there's been a win. Occasionally, riders may have a glass of red wine at night to help them relax, but usually only the one. For any serious bike rider, the advice is to keep alcohol to a minimum, especially around key training sessions, competitions and events.

MICRONUTRIENTS: THE 'GLOW NUTRIENTS'

Micronutrients are vitamins, minerals and electrolytes and I consider these the 'glow nutrients'. We need them for health, well-being and the smooth running of the body.

Vitamins

Vitamins are a collection of complex carbon-based molecular compounds that have a wide range of physiological functions. They are classified into two groups based on their solubility: fat-soluble and water-soluble vitamins. Fat-soluble vitamins (A, D, E and K) can be readily stored in the body so that they are available when needed. If consumed to excess, however, they can build up to harmful levels. Water-soluble vitamins (B group and C) are not generally stored, and any excess intake is excreted in urine. They can still, however, be toxic in excessive amounts.

Minerals

Along with the macronutrients and vitamins in the food we eat, we also consume small amounts of inorganic compounds such as metal and non-metal ions. An example is table salt which contains both sodium chloride and potassium iodide. These compounds dissolve in the gut, releasing ions which are crucial to cell function and water balance in the body. The iodide ion is needed for the production of the hormone thyroxine.

Some minerals are required in relatively large amounts, over 100 milligrams, and these are referred to as the macrominerals. There are seven of them: calcium, phosphorus, chlorine, potassium, sulphur, sodium and magnesium. The microminerals, iron, copper, zinc and fluorine, are needed in milligram amounts. And the trace minerals include iodine, selenium, vanadium, chromium, manganese, cobalt, nickel, molybdenum and tin and are needed in microgram amounts. All of these minerals are essential to optimal body function and performance.

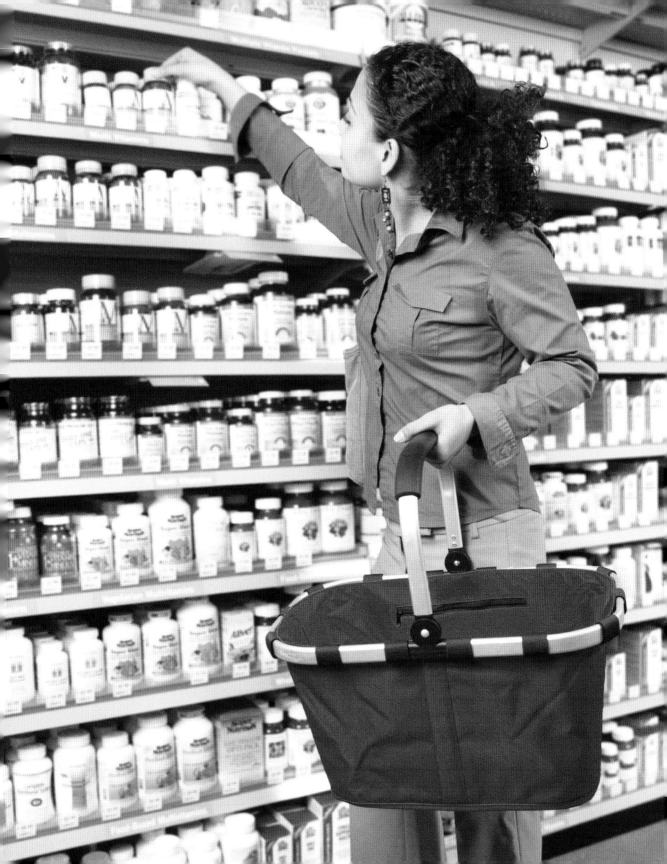

DO I NEED TO TAKE A MULTIVITAMIN AND MULTI-MINERAL?

There is considerable debate as to whether taking a multivitamin or multi-mineral has any real value. From my point of view, if we have a good, well-balanced diet we should be getting all of the nutrients we need. The problem is we do not always know exactly how many nutrients we are getting from our food and it's also difficult to fully assess an individual's requirements. So even though I like riders to get their nutrients from their diet at times of high physical demand, I think taking a simple multivitamin or mineral that provides up to 100 per cent of the dietary recommended value can be a sensible, prudent approach.

There are, however, a couple of exceptions regarding supplementation and sport, notably vitamin D and iron. Over recent years we have developed a greater understanding of the issues of insufficient vitamin D levels. The body can synthesise vitamin D using sunlight. However, in recent years, partly due to a greater awareness of the dangers of sun overexposure, many people are not spending enough time in the sun so are not synthesising vitamin D to the right level. Vitamin D has many physiological functions, including an integral role in bone health, and it is also important for the immune and nervous system. Many athletes in the Northern Hemisphere will take a vitamin D supplement from October to March, when there is less sunshine. Currently it is believed that there is little risk in taking a vitamin D supplement during this time and potentially some benefit. It is not clear exactly how sub-optimal vitamin D levels directly affect health and performance except subtly compromising the immune system and recovery. The current recommended upper dosage of vitamin D is 400 iu (100 micrograms) per day.

Iron can also sometimes be an issue. Hard training can cause a more rapid turnover of iron. This can lead to low iron levels, anaemia and associated symptoms such as fatigue, reduced performance and poor recovery. The main issue with iron supplementation is how much you absorb and the negative side effects it can have on the digestive system, such as constipation. If you suspect that low iron levels are negatively affecting your cycling, seek advice on supplementation from a medical professional.

Water

With the human body composed of approximately 70 per cent water, it should be no surprise that you need to keep it topped up with fluid to perform optimally. On Grand Tours we'd weigh our riders daily and take urine samples to keep track of their hydration levels. Whether you're training, tackling a sportive, riding a multi-day epic or racing, if you're not keeping hydrated, you'll be compromising your performance, limiting training gains and prolonging the recovery process. Hydration, both on and off the bike, is a key area that we'll cover in detail later in the book.

'OLD SCHOOL' VS MODERN GRAND TOUR DIET

Meal	'Old school' 1950s diet	Modern diet
Pre-stage breakfast	Steak, bread, cheese	Porridge, omelette, fruit smoothie
On the bike	Panini, cakes, water	Energy bars, rice cakes, panini, gels, sports drinks
Post-ride recovery	Sandwich	Protein/carbohydrate recovery drink (providing approximately 20 g protein and 40 g of carbohydrate), followed by fresh rice cooked in rice cooker
Dinner	Salads, chicken, pasta, vegetables, bread	Salads, chicken, mashed sweet potato, vegetables, vegetable juice

KITCHEN ESSENTIALS

There are three bits of kitchen equipment that I wouldn't be without. As well as planning the diets of Grand Tour winners, I was also responsible, along with the team chef, for delivering them. During our reconnaissance of the opening stages of the 2014 Tour de France with Team Sky, these were my must-haves for feeding the team and I'd strongly recommend you get them for your kitchen too.

Rice cooker: A very simple piece of kit with prices ranging from £15–£60 ($20–$80). I get through loads of these, not because they break, but because I give them away to riders! My favourite one at the moment is the Tefal Multi Cooker – it can be used for rice, soups, porridge and lots more.

Slow cooker: I use this nearly every day. The great thing is you can throw everything in, switch it on, go out for a six-hour ride and come home to great food. I have used these a lot to feed riders after the Spring Classics on the bus. I don't have a preference for these, but the one I have at the moment is a Crock Pot that's nearly four years old.

Food processor/juicer: There are loads on the market, but I love my Thermomix and I have taken it all over Europe. The great thing with it is that, not only can you accurately weigh out the ingredients, you can cook at controlled temperatures and have a very powerful liquidiser; it really does do it all. The main drawback, however, is the cost. At about £900 ($1,200), I don't give these away to riders!

KNOWLEDGE TO TAKE AWAY

- **'Go Nutrients'** *Carbohydrates, fats and proteins are the nutrients that fuel activity, growth and repair; they're what make you go.*

- **'Glow Nutrients'** *Vitamins and minerals are necessary for health, well-being and optimal function; they're what make you glow.*

- **Alcohol** *Empty calories that get stored as fat, reduce recovery and have a diuretic effect; best avoided or kept to a minimum around key training sessions, competitions and events.*

- **Supplements** *If you're eating a balanced and healthy diet, there should be no need for general multivitamins and multi-minerals. However, if you're training hard, travelling or putting your body under unusual stress, taking a quality product can be a wise choice.*

- **Vitamin D and Iron** *Supplementation of these nutrients can be beneficial and necessary for some endurance athletes, but possible issues should first be identified with a blood test.*

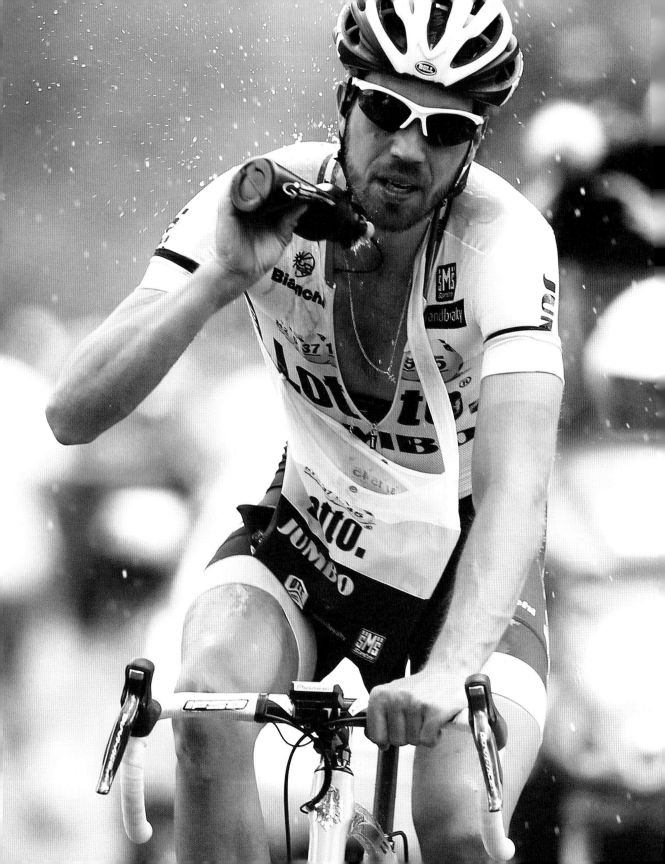

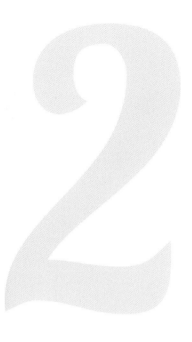

GUT HEALTH: WORKING FROM THE INSIDE OUT

Before talking about how best to fuel your training and racing, it's essential to take a look inside and tackle the neglected area of gut function and health. If you haven't got a healthy gut, you can be taking in the best fuel, at exactly the right times and in the optimum quantities, but you simply won't perform. It's like having a car with a blocked fuel line. You're putting the fuel in, but not enough is getting through to the engine for it to fire up to anywhere near its maximum potential.

Endurance sports, especially a three-week Grand Tour or a heavy block of training, are incredibly stressful on the body and so on the gut too. When I was working as a clinical dietician in the mid-nineties with immune compromised patients suffering from conditions such as cancer, HIV and AIDS, optimising gut health was a key part of their treatment. With hard training cyclists, because gut health is directly linked to our immune system, I've found the stresses to be similar. Factor in additional potential stresses to the gut, such as exercising in the heat, the inevitable muck from the road spraying onto water bottles, large quantities of highly acidic sports drinks and the differing mineral content of water abroad, and it's easy to see why gut health is such an issue for riders. Some of these variables we can control and others we can't, but I've always prioritised making my riders' guts as healthy and robust as possible and you should try to do the same.

Martijn Keizer of Lotto NL–Jumbo team attempts to cool down in the hot conditions during the 2016 Tour Down Under

GUT ANATOMY

Mouth

The first stage in the digestive process is chewing and forming a bolus of food that can be swallowed. Enzymes, such as salivary amylase, are also introduced at this point, which starts the chemical digestion. You can make a real difference to digestion and gut health by simply taking the time to chew your food properly. Saliva is also an important part of the immune system, producing antibodies such as IgA and antimicrobial compounds. Having a prolonged dry mouth may therefore compromise your immune system, so keep sipping from that bidon.

Stomach and small intestine

The stomach is simply a big churning muscular sack full of acid that breaks food down mechanically and chemically.

Gut anatomy

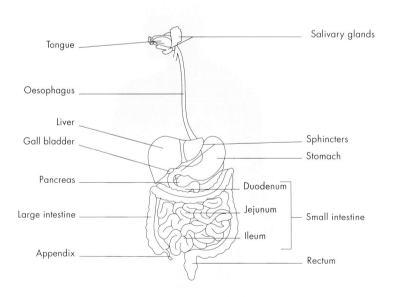

Tongue — Salivary glands

Oesophagus

Liver

Gall bladder — Sphincters — Stomach

Pancreas — Duodenum

Large intestine — Jejunum — Small intestine

Ileum

Appendix — Rectum

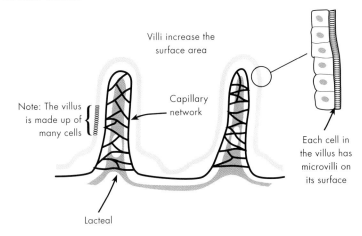

Villi increase the surface area

Note: The villus is made up of many cells

Capillary network

Each cell in the villus has microvilli on its surface

Lacteal

The small intestine is the key area of the gut where most of the digestion and absorption of nutrients takes place. It's covered by millions of finger-like projections called villi, which increase the surface area. A healthy small intestine is also densely populated by good bacteria, also known as microbiota or gut flora, which aid the digestive process. For the small intestine to function optimally, it has to have an alkaline pH, but the content emptying into it from the stomach is highly acidic. Pancreatic enzymes raise the pH, but aiding this alkalisation of the lower intestine is one of the keys to gut health.

Large intestine

Some further absorption of nutrients takes place in the large intestine (colon), but this area of the gut is primarily concerned with the uptake of water, drawing it out of the passing mass of largely indigestible food matter. The large intestine is also a very important part of the immune system, with its good bacteria playing a key role. Fibre plays a really important role in the large intestine, helping to form the bulk of a stool, keeping it soft. Some fibre, known as prebiotics, is a fuel for the gut bacteria. Most fibre-containing foods contains a mix of both soluble and insoluble fibre. Typically the insoluble fibre is found in the skins of fruit and vegetables and the bran portion of wholegrains whereas the insoluble fibre is found in the flesh.

Rectum

Waste material from the digestive process constitutes the faecal mass, which is stored in the rectum prior to excretion via the anus. If your digestive system is healthy, you should be having at least two bowel movements per day; if not, you may not be getting enough fibre.

POOR GUT HEALTH ISSUES AND CAUSES

The majority of sporting gut health issues can normally be traced back to those finger-like projections, the villi, in your small intestine being compromised and not functioning correctly. If you suffer from excessive wind, characterised by discomfort and bloating, constipation or diarrhoea, have big fluctuations in energy levels or excessively crave sugary foods and drinks, you could well have an issue with your gut health. Many cyclists will shrug off these symptoms; I've heard riders talk and laugh about 'gel guts' after a ride, but it's not normal, not unavoidable and will be compromising your performance.

The very nature of sport puts extra stress on the digestive system. As we exercise the blood flow which supplies your digestive system is redirected to our hard-working peripheral muscles. This means that there is less blood supply, which not only affects digestion but the reduction in blood can affect gut health and in extreme cases leads to damage. Additionally, exercise increases our core temperature, which can also reduce gut function.

Gastrointestinal infections

Any gastrointestinal infection or upset, such as food poisoning, which results in vomiting and diarrhoea, will have a negative effect on the villi. Unfortunately, endurance training can compromise the immune system and, if you're racing or training abroad, you'll also be exposed to new bacteria that your body isn't familiar with. This is why pro cyclists are so diligent about hygiene. Always wash your hands well, use antibacterial gel and make sure you keep your water bottles spotlessly clean.

Training

Training is stressful on the body and on the gut. Although you probably won't be putting your body through the wringer in the same way a Grand Tour rider will, in many ways it can be tougher for an amateur rider. You've got work and family stress, and, if you pile training on top of that, it's a lot to ask of your body. Riding for hours in the heat can also compromise the villi, so, although those summer rides and warm weather training camps might feel great, your gut is going to be struggling.

pH levels

As I've already mentioned, an alkaline lower intestine is optimum, but the content emptying into it from the stomach is highly acidic. Under normal circumstances our body copes with this, but hard training and racing isn't normal. Most sports drinks are highly acidic and you may get through many bottles on a long ride. Also, the stress of training and racing causes the stomach to release more of its own acid. By adding to the acidity in your stomach in these ways, it's tougher for the lower intestine to achieve its necessary alkaline state.

Having an occasional bottle of sports drink should not be a problem and some people can consume large quantities of them with no effect but some people are more sensitive. We're all individuals, so it's vital to know your own body. There are now companies that make neutral pH sports drinks, which a lot of riders find useful and easier on their stomachs, so you may want to try these.

Although it initially made me unpopular with some of the

riders, I've always implemented a policy of not giving out cans of cola after races or training, despite the fact that many of them really crave one. These drinks have a really low pH and having one when the body is stressed undermines all the healthy gut health strategies that we've put in place. The only time we use cola is an occasional small can in the feed bag in hard stages as a little 'pick me up'. I'd advise cutting cola and similar carbonated highly sugared drinks out of your diet as much as possible.

Intolerances

If you've suffered from a gastrointestinal infection in the past, you'll know that lactose-rich foods such as milk and cheese exacerbate the situation. This doesn't mean you've necessarily got a lactose intolerance, it's just means that, under stress, your gut can't handle it as well. Hard training puts your body under stress, so, under those circumstances, you might be best to avoid it too. The same can apply to gluten and wheat, and if you have toast for breakfast, a sandwich for lunch and pasta for dinner, it can just be wheat overload, so it's no surprise you might be up half the night with indigestion. Again this doesn't mean that you're necessarily gluten intolerant, it might just mean you need to reduce or cut it out when you're putting in the miles. I have worked with several professional riders who have started with the team saying that they were gluten intolerant. Then, having followed a healthy gut regime for a while, I'd see them happily eating pasta and bread with the other riders. I'd remind them that they'd told me they were gluten intolerant and they'd say that it had just cleared up and they no longer had any issues! I'll talk more about both gluten- and lactose-free diets in Chapter 10.

Bad vs good bacteria

Our lower intestine should have a rich flora of good bacteria which aids digestion. Much of the fibre we eat, referred to as 'prebiotic', fuels these good bacteria and is one of the reasons why fibre from fruit and vegetables is so important. However, if gut conditions aren't optimal, conditions can occur which are more conducive to the proliferation of bad bacteria. These bacteria ferment the fibre, producing toxins, gas and reducing villi function.

Leaky gut

Each individual villi is separated by a protein barrier. If the villi are damaged or 'stressed', these protein barriers can break down and gaps may appear. Toxins from the the small intestine then 'leak' into the bloodstream, leading to further complications and stress for the body.

PRO STORY: SOME RIDERS ARE LIKE BILLY GOATS

We're all individuals with differing degrees of gut sensitivity and robustness. Some riders I've worked with, such as Sir Bradley Wiggins, are like billy goats and can eat almost anything, whether on or off the bike, with no negative effects. Some of the concoctions we gave Wiggins to try were unbelievable and he just tolerated them. At the other end of the spectrum, some riders had incredibly sensitive guts. One particular rider would struggle to race over more than 200 km without having to stop for a comfort break. We developed a pH neutral sports drink for him and also gels using natural fruit juice, which were far easier on his stomach. We also looked at his race food. If you're eating two bars an hour, that's a lot of fibre being consumed, which will produce a lot of faecal mass. We produced rice cakes which were 100 per cent digestible and allowed him to fuel properly without having to worry about stopping. Similar rice cakes are now a staple race food for most pro riders.

GUT PROTECTION PACKAGE

If you tend to suffer from digestive issues on the bike or regularly display any of the symptoms described previously, you should be looking to enhance your gut health as your first nutritional step in improving your cycling performance. Even if you think your gut is healthy, if you're planning a big training block or are travelling to train or race abroad, giving your gut health a boost is a really good idea.

If you've had a gastrointestinal infection, a bad stomach reaction or have recently undergone a course of antibiotics, you should follow my gut rehab plan.

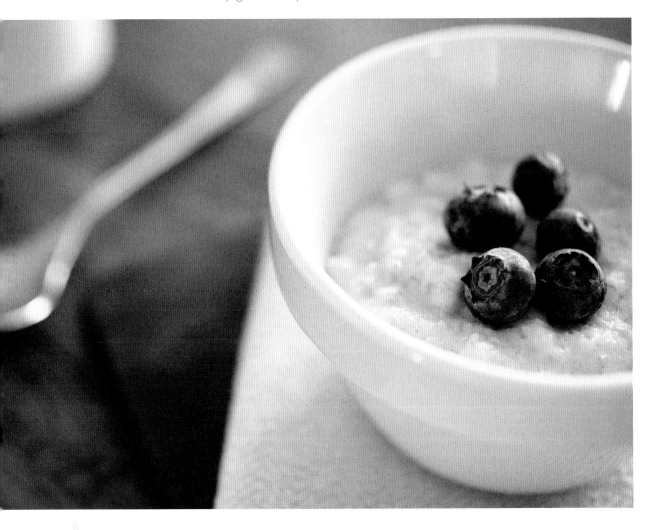

Gut rehab plan

I use this plan to help riders to recover from gut disturbances and have used it with a huge variety of other athletes from a range of sports. I've even had to use it with athletes who picked up gastroenteritis at the World Championships and it allowed them to go on and win a world title. It's important, however, that, if you regularly suffer from gastrointestinal issues, you consult with a doctor to check if there are any underlying medical conditions. You should follow the guidelines for three to five days, but should notice improvements within 24 hours.

- Avoid wheat and gluten. Even if you're not sensitive or intolerant to gluten, if your digestive system is compromised or you're under particular stress, it can be an irritant on the small intestine. Bread, pasta and biscuits should all be cut out and should be substituted with porridge oats, rice, potatoes and alternative grains, such as quinoa.
- Avoid high sources of lactose. Again, like gluten, when people have gastric issues they often have a mild temporary lactose intolerance. Cut out cow's milk and other dairy products, such as cheese and butter. Replace with soya or rice milk. You can eat up to 100 g of natural yoghurt each day as the manufacturing process breaks down a large proportion of the lactose.
- You should opt for easily digested protein sources, such as chicken, fish and eggs, and avoid red meat. Cut out known gut irritants, such as coffee, tea, high-sugar foods, fruit juices (because of the high levels of fermentable sugars) and alcohol. Fruit teas and herbal infusions are okay if you want a hot drink.

An example meal plan would be:
- **Breakfast:** Porridge made with soya milk, topped with blueberries, an optional scoop of protein powder (you can mix this in with the porridge and some brands even contain beneficial probiotics) and a yoghurt. A glass of vegetable juice

or 'energised greens' (see page 172)

- **On the bike:** Rice cakes (see pages 112–113)
- **Lunch:** Salmon, quinoa and rice, steamed carrots and tomatoes
- **Dinner:** Chicken breast, baked sweet potato, fresh salad including tomatoes and a glass of vegetable juice or 'energised greens'
- **Pre-bedtime snack:** Natural yoghurt (not exceeding 100 g total for day) or a serving of protein powder.

EASILY-DIGESTIBLE DIET

We're constantly being told to eat five a day and, although fruit and vegetables are essential for a healthy diet and give the good bacteria the fuel they need, fibrous food is a real load on the digestive system if you're training hard. It can end up sitting in the gut fermenting and contributes to large amounts of faecal mass. Vegetable juices and energised greens (an easy-to-use blend of nutrient dense greens) are a brilliant way to get the nutrients and soluble fibre without the gut-stressing bulk of whole vegetables and salads. Eat plenty of highly-digestible protein, such as chicken and fish, and, on the bike, eat snacks such as rice cakes rather than fibre-filled bars, bananas or dried fruit. From a carbohydrate perspective, rice (particularly basmati rice) is really easily digestible and, because of the high water content, can help with hydration.

Probiotics

Probiotics are the good bacteria in your gut and, by taking products such as Yakult, Actimel and even some protein powders, you can reinforce your own populations. Active yoghurts and fermented foods can also add to the probiotics. There's a bit of controversy as to how many actually make it through the harsh environment of the stomach, but clinical research has shown that their use can boost immune function and reduce conditions such as chest infections. It is believed that this is achieved by helping to protect the villi and reduce 'leaky gut'.

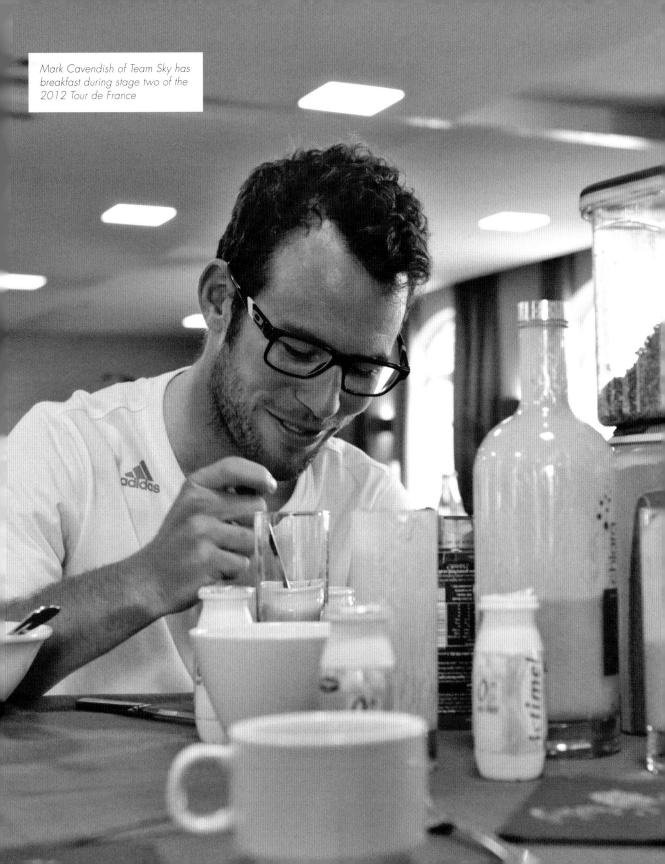

Mark Cavendish of Team Sky has breakfast during stage two of the 2012 Tour de France

The latest thinking regarding taking probiotics (good bacteria) is to have various strains and from various sources. Fermented products, such as live yoghurt, provide an excellent source of active good bacteria and foods such as pickles can help support the probiotics. Kefir is a fermented milk drink that is gaining popularity. Originating from the Caucasus Mountains, it combines both yeasts and bacteria that work together symbiotically. The fermented drink produced provides multiple strains of probiotics and the yeasts break down the lactose in the milk so that people with lactose sensitivity are usually okay with kefir drinks.

There are many products on the market that provide probiotics. These can be useful when travelling or if you are taking a course of antibiotics and trying to maintain gut health.

Supplements

Colostrum is the milk produced by cows during the first 24 hours following birth. It's high in growth and immune factors and is excellent for helping to protect the villi. The dosage for this is about 10–20 g a day, usually taken after exercise.

Glutamine is an amino acid which research has shown to be beneficial for recovery both for sporting performance and in clinical settings such as burns wards. Along with protective and restorative properties for the gut, it can also be used as a fuel. A daily dosage of 5–15 g/day may provide benefits.

Having adequate amounts of omega-3 oils may also help the gut. You can achieve this by eating oily fish, such as sardines and mackerel, but often people will use a supplement for convenience. Milled flax and chia seeds provide a suitable vegetarian option and can easily be added to smoothies or sprinkled on food. You can find more information on omega-3 oils and other supplements in Chapter 9.

ENHANCE ALKALINITY AND REDUCE ACIDITY

The vegetable juices that I'll be recommending and giving you recipes for later in the book are great for creating a more alkaline small intestine. Cutting down on dairy, processed food and red meat will also help you to reduce acidity. Look out for sports drinks with a lower pH, and cut out all carbonated soft drinks as they are highly acidic. Flat cola can be great, however, to get you through the final stretch of a one-off event such as an Ironman triathlon, but, if you're wanting to race or train for multiple consecutive days, it's a big no.

CUT OUT OR REDUCE KNOWN IRRITANTS

Alcohol, especially concentrated spirits, is an irritant to the gut. A beer or a glass of wine won't hurt, but avoid overdoing it. We all know how we feel on Christmas Day after eating and drinking too much; it feels awful and is incredibly stressful for the whole body. Caffeine in tea or coffee is another irritant. Again, moderation is fine, but take it easy.

LOW-RESIDUE DIET

When I was working as a clinical dietician in the NHS we'd use a low-residue diet to reduce faecal mass prior to bowel surgery. When I started working with athletes, I applied this knowledge to weight management as faecal mass can account for up to 2 kg of dead weight. Also, less faecal mass means lower digestive stress so it can be helpful if you suffer from digestive issues during events.

One potential issue with removing the fibre is a reduction in some of the prebiotics which are used as a fuel by the gut bacteria. Therefore, the low-residue diet is not recommended to be used long term. Also, anyone following this plan should top up with fresh vegetable juice, ready-made vegetable juices such as V8, energised greens or prune juice.

A low-residue diet simply involves following a highly digestible but extremely monotonous diet in the final build-up to an event. You'd want to start it three days before, so if your event was on the Saturday, you'd begin it on the Wednesday evening.

An example meal plan would be:
- **Breakfast:** White basmati rice and an omelette
- **Lunch:** White basmati rice with chicken or fish
- **Dinner:** Repeat lunch with natural yoghurt for desert and maybe a protein shake before bed.

Because this is a pre-event diet, it's not at all energy restrictive so, although you're eating very simple and easy-to-digest meals, total calorie consumption isn't limited. Different riders respond in a variety of ways to it, so it's something to try in training. Some lose significant weight, feel super-energised and ride half a Grand Tour on it, whereas others don't lose any and feel a bit flat.

Interestingly, I've had lots of positive feedback from riders tackling long-time trials as they feel it makes holding an aerodynamic position more comfortable. Even Great Britain's cycling team pursuit team liked it for this reason.

KNOWLEDGE TO TAKE AWAY

- **Healthy gut** There's no point thinking about optimal nutrition if your gut isn't functioning well. It's like having a car with a blocked fuel line.

- **Causes** There are multiple stressors on our digestive system and causes of poor gut health. Work through them all to achieve optimal gut health.

- **Solutions** Give your gut a helping hand by cutting out irritants and consider using some key supplements.

- **Individuals** We're all different. Some of us have sensitive digestive systems whereas others can eat almost anything. However, even riders with very sensitive stomachs, by carefully managing their gut health, can take on the toughest events.

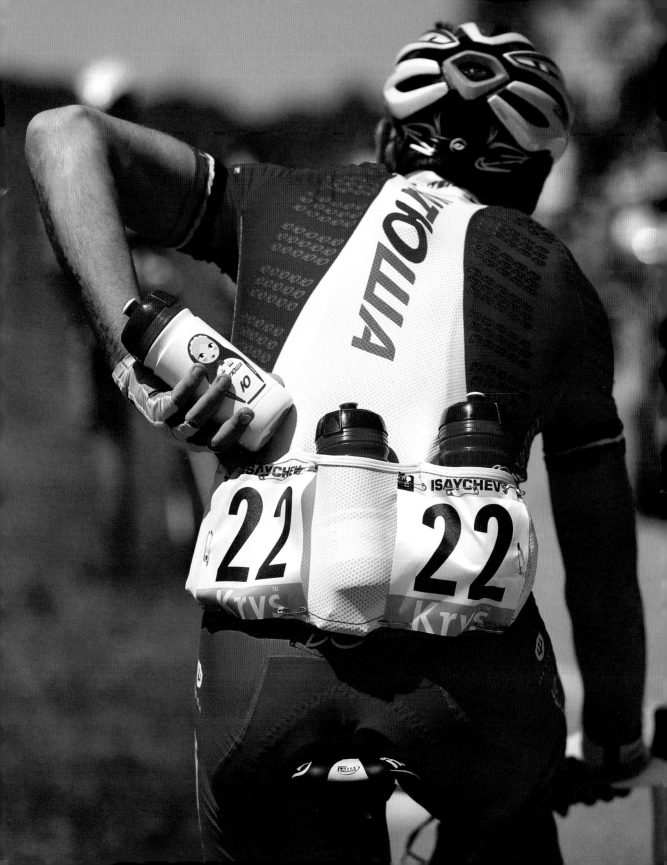

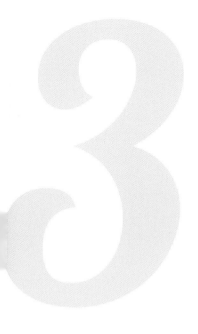

OPTIMAL HYDRATION

Before talking about the food to fuel your cycling, it's important to ensure that you're optimally hydrated. Our bodies are made up of about 70 per cent water and every one of our individual cells works on a finely maintained balance between fluid on the inside of the cell and on the outside. Think of the amoeba, which, because of having a permeable membrane, has to maintain a careful balance between the fluid and salts (electrolytes) inside it and the water outside. If the concentration of electrolytes in the cell is too high, fluid will enter the cell from the outside to redress the balance. Without this mechanism and the watery environment surrounding the amoeba, it wouldn't be able to survive. We evolved from single-celled organisms into a much more complex multicellular organisms, but our cells, like the amoeba's, still depend on this water and electrolyte balance to maintain homeostasis, their balance, and function.

The topic of hydration for athletic performance has recently attracted a fair amount of controversy, and, with various sources misreporting and misinterpreting research, it's understandable that many people are confused. The problem is that, for years, some sports drink manufacturers have sponsored research that has encouraged people to drink sugar-laden sports drinks when it simply isn't necessary. How many times have you seen someone at the gym doing 30 minutes of fairly low-intensity exercise and diligently sipping at sports drink? They're probably consuming more calories from that drink than they're using during their workout. At times, we have also been over prescriptive regarding drinking frequency during exercise. There is currently a bit of a backlash against both sport drinks and the recommended rate of fluid consumption during exercise. You have some voices recommending to only drink when thirsty and others saying that thirst is an unreliable indicator of hydration level. In this chapter, I draw on my experience and explain what hydration strategy I feel is most

Vladimir Isaychev of Team Katusha collects water bottles for his teammates during the 2014 Tour de France

appropriate for both professional and amateur cyclists. Along with cycling, I have worked with a number of other sports, including golf, swimming, football, boxing and sailing, and have found the hydration requirements for optimal performance to be significantly different. A generic hydration strategy that covers all sports just isn't, in my experience, realistic as all activities have unique demands.

Studies in endurance exercise have shown that surprisingly low fluid losses can significantly affect your ability to ride. A 2 per cent drop in body weight due to sweating (1.6 kg for an 80 kg rider) will impair performance noticeably, 4 per cent will decrease your capacity for muscular work, and, with a 5 per cent drop, heat exhaustion can become an issue and your capacity for work will drop by up to 30 per cent. Hit 7 per cent and you'll start experiencing hallucinations and, at 10 per cent, circulatory collapse, heatstroke and even death become possibilities. Not only does this dehydration potentially affect performance, but we can also see changes in the fluid spaces in the brain which affects cognitive ability and concentration.

Another key area where hydration impacts on cycling performance is recovery. If you're dehydrated, recovery will be significantly compromised. For cyclists, whether riding a Grand Tour, on a training camp or simply putting in back-to-back sessions, this is a serious consideration.

To see why these drops in performances occur, we can look at the body as a whole, but to understand the fluid in our bodies better we should break it down into compartments: intracellular and extracellular fluid. Simply put, intracellular fluid is found within our cells and extracellular fluid outside of them. The extracellular fluid can be again subcategorized: it includes the plasma volume, which is the fluid in the blood carrying our blood cells, and the interstitial fluid, which bathes and surrounds the cells of our body's tissues.

When we ride, even in cool conditions, we are constantly

losing fluid through sweating and breathing. The more we exercise the more we sweat, breathe harder and the more fluid we lose. Sweating is an essential process because, as the sweat evaporates, it takes heat energy from the body and helps to keep us cool. However, as we sweat, we lose fluid from our body and, if we do not replace it, we end up with a deficit. If not corrected, this can lead to dehydration, which means more concentrated body fluid compartments and a reduced ability to regulate our temperature. In severe dehydration, cells will actually die (think of our amoebas as a pond drying up). Mild dehydration results in a reduced blood plasma, leading to a number of knock-on effects, including decreased sweat rate, heat dissipation (reduced ability to cool down) and digestive function. Your core temperature will increase and so too will the rate of muscle glycogen use. The net effect of these physiological changes is that your body has to work increasingly harder to maintain the same effort. Sooner rather than later this increased workload become unsustainable and performance sharply drops.

HYDRATION OFF THE BIKE

Even on days when you're not riding, you should still be aware of keeping well hydrated. Our bodies function far better if hydrated, with energy levels and digestive function especially compromised if we allow ourselves to become dehydrated. I have seen many athletes with chronic mild dehydration, which not only affects athletic performance but focus and work performance too. For many of us, work itself provides a hydration challenge as we often work in an air-conditioned environment, which can increase the risk of dehydration.

Weigh yourself daily, especially if you're already fairly lean, as sudden significant drops in weight probably suggest that you should up your fluid intake. This daily weighing is routine on most pro teams and, in conjunction with urine colour charts (see

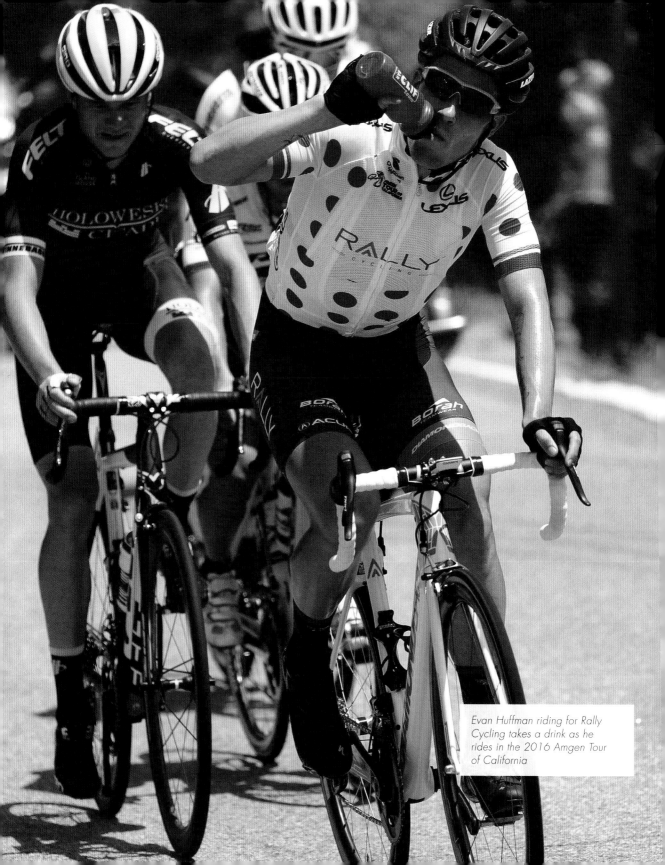

Evan Huffman riding for Rally Cycling takes a drink as he rides in the 2016 Amgen Tour of California

Appendix 1, page 228), is a great tool for monitoring hydration. Along with monitoring your hydration level, try to drink 2–3 l of fluids a day, whether you're riding or not. Fruit and vegetable juices, sports drinks and water all count towards this target, but alcohol, tea, coffee and sugar-laden soft drinks don't.

On the night before a big ride, if you've been monitoring and keeping on top of your hydration, there should be no need to drink excessively the night before or in the hours leading up to a ride. If you drink excessive amounts in a forlorn hope of playing catch-up in terms of hydration, you'll only succeed in guaranteeing early and numerous 'comfort breaks'. In the two hours leading up to a long ride, tough training session or race, sip on 500–750 ml of isotonic (see below) carbohydrate sports fuel to ensure optimal hydration and fully stocked up energy reserves.

HYDRATION ON THE BIKE
How much to drink on the bike

We are all individuals and we lose fluid at different rates so it's useful to get to know your own requirements. A simple way to test this is to do a sweat test on the turbo. Having hydrated well during the day, weigh yourself in the nude and note your weight down. With the room at about 20 °C (68°F) and ensuring you have adequate airflow from a fan, ride at your normal sportive or racing intensity for 60 minutes. For a ride of this length you shouldn't need to consume any water, but, if you do, ensure you note down how much you consume. As soon as you finish, strip, towel off any sweat from your skin and weigh yourself again. Work out your fluid loss using the following formula:

Nude weight before ride (g) + fluid consumed during ride (ml) − Nude weight after ride (g) = fluid loss during ride (ml)

Obviously the results will vary according to weather conditions and riding intensity and you may want to perform several tests to get a range of readings, but it will still give you a good idea of how much you sweat during cycling. Most riders will find that they will typically lose 500–1000 ml per hour. If you're at the upper end of this range, it might not be practical or necessary to try and replace it all, but you should aim for a minimum of 65–75 per cent.

Timing drinking on the bike

For any long ride, you should be aiming to hit your hydration target right from the start with regular sips from your bottles every 10–15 minutes. Even among the pros, some riders are better at remembering to drink than others, but if you tend to forget, setting an alarm is a good idea. Don't forget your recovery drink at the end of a long ride either. No matter how diligent you've been with your hydration, especially on a hot day, you're likely to be dehydrated and, as well as providing the protein and carbohydrate to kick-start your recovery, the fluids and electrolytes that a recovery drink provide are essential.

What to drink on the bike

Exactly what and when you drink on the bike is affected by numerous variables, such as the intensity and length of the ride, the climatic conditions and your individual needs. It's hard therefore to give concrete guidelines and you should use these recommendations as a starting point and, by experimenting in training and under different conditions, find the hydration strategy that works best for you.

For rides of under 60 minutes, plain water is fine, but on longer rides, water on its own won't deliver any energy, can cause you to feel bloated and will reduce your desire to drink well before fluid losses have been replaced. For longer rides, therefore, you'll need to add electrolytes and carbohydrates. This can be in the form of food: a medium banana, for example, will provide about 30 g of carbohydrate and some electrolytes, in particular potassium. Electrolytes are salts that include sodium, potassium, calcium and magnesium. They are lost in sweat, but are essential for normal cellular function so have to be replaced.

Most commercially available sports drinks have a careful balance of electrolytes, but, if you're not wanting to use drinking to take on calories, effervescent electrolyte tablets without any carbohydrates are also available.

For longer rides, it makes sense to combine drinking with calorie intake: 500 ml of typical sports drink mixed at 4 per cent (4 g of carbohydrate per 100 ml of water) will give you 20 g of carbohydrate, which makes for an easy way to contribute to your total energy requirement (see pages 147–149).

The concentration of typical sports drinks can vary from about 4 to 8 per cent carbohydrate. Some riders, however, prefer to take all carbohydrate in the form of liquid and will take drinks as high as 20 per cent (100 g per 500 ml) concentration, which they will consume in conjunction with a second bottle containing plain water. Although this can work well for some riders, it takes a lot of training for the gut to be able to cope with that concentration of carbohydrate. This is definitely not a tactic to try for the first time on an important ride.

Most sports drinks will contain a blend of carbohydrates combining maltodextrin and simple sugars, such as glucose and fructose. Cheaper sports drinks will contain a higher proportion of sucrose (table sugar). Maltodextrin is composed of a long chain of glucose molecules joined together. This structure reduces the 'osmotic pressure', typically making the drinks kinder on your stomach. The osmotic pressure of a solution is largely determined by its concentration and, if high, will pull water out of your blood into your gut to dilute it. As it can't be absorbed until it has been diluted, it sits in your gut, sloshing around and making you feel unwell. The idea of mixing the types of carbohydrate is to have multiple carbohydrate sources. As glucose is absorbed via a particular transporter in the gut and fructose a different one, the idea is that, by taking advantage of the two systems, you can increase absorption and delivery. Some sports drinks also contain protein and/or BCAAs (Branch Chain Amino Acids), but, although

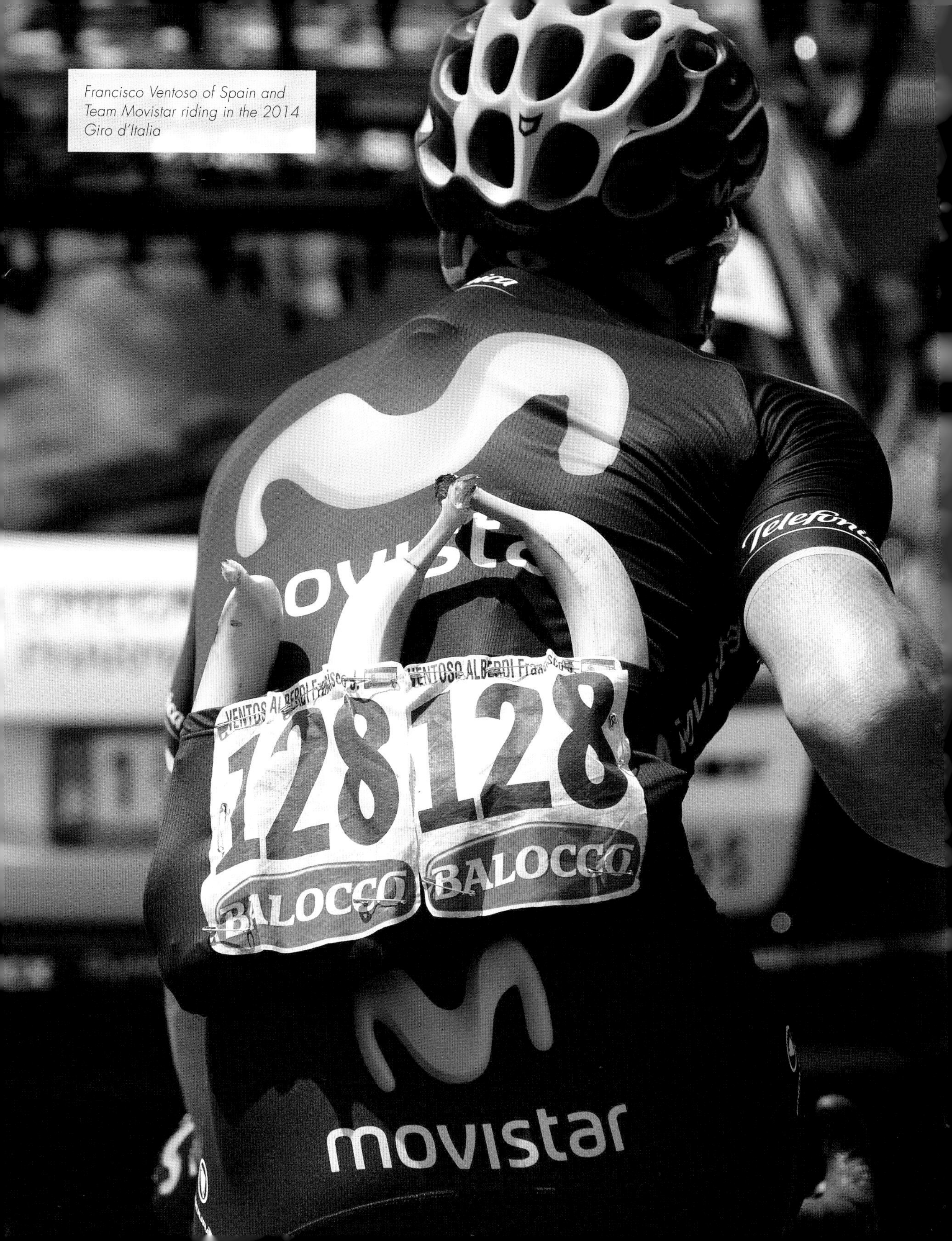

Francisco Ventoso of Spain and Team Movistar riding in the 2014 Giro d'Italia

there is some evidence of benefits during endurance activities, the jury is still out. However, for carbohydrate-fasted rides, which we'll discuss later in the book (see pages 106–109), the use of a protein-based drink is definitely beneficial.

My preferred sports drink for riders is pretty simple: each serving should provide 20 g of carbohydrate with 15 g from maltodextrin and 5 g from fructose. It should contain a balance of electrolytes, including sodium, potassium and magnesium, have a neutral pH and have a mild flavour. This type of drink is ideal for the high volume usage required by cyclists, and this drinks profile is what you should be looking for when selecting a sports drink. Many commercially available drinks tick a couple of these boxes, but there are only a few that tick all, especially the crucial neutral pH one. These sports drinks are definitely worth seeking out though, especially if you tend to suffer from gastrointestinal (GI) issues when riding.

As all sports drinks contain slightly differing ingredients, it's important that you try them in training to find one that suits you. If you're taking part in a sportive or race, find out which manufacturer is supplying the feed stations and try their product beforehand to check you get on with it. If you're unable to do this, bag up your own preferred brand in measured quantities and just mix it with the water provided. Don't gamble on untested nutritional products as digestive distress is guaranteed to ruin your ride.

Don't forget that food can provide fluid too. Foods such as the rice cakes are cooked rice so not only provide carbohydrates but a decent amount of liquid too. If you choose to just eat dry foods, such as energy bars, you'll need to drink more. Food can also provide electrolytes. Bananas, for example, are an excellent source of potassium.

When you dissolve your sports drink powder in water, the concentration of the solution will affect how easily it passes out of your gut, how quickly it hydrates you and how well it quenches your thirst. Osmolarity is a measure of the number of dissolved molecules in a solution, including electrolytes and carbohydrates. Blood typically has an osmolarity of around 300 mOsm/kg and so a solution with a similar osmolarity is said to be isotonic ('iso' meaning the same). If the osmolarity is higher, it's hypertonic, and if it's lower, it's hypotonic.

ISOTONIC

Isotonic drinks are most relevant to endurance sports as they strike a perfect balance between replacing fluids, supplying carbohydrates and electrolytes and keeping your thirst stimulated. If you follow the mixing guidelines on most sports drinks, the 6–8 per cent solution will typically be isotonic.

HYPOTONIC

Plain water, or very weak orange squash, is hypotonic. It'll replace lost fluids very quickly, but won't deliver significant energy or electrolytes. Also, as previously mentioned, hypotonic drinks will often reduce your desire to drink more before you've replaced adequate fluids and leave you feeling bloated.

HYPERTONIC

Hypertonic drinks are strong solutions of carbohydrates that can be used for higher calorie intakes. As I've already mentioned, some riders will have one bottle loaded up with an extremely strong carbohydrate solution and use this in conjunction with plain water in their other bottle. You can also try this approach for lower intensity winter rides, where you won't be sweating heavily. They will leave your stomach fairly slowly though and, as they can also cause gastric distress, should be thoroughly tried in training first.

HYDRATION IN THE COLD

Riders tend to drink a lot less on colder days, but still sweat and lose fluids. I've seen this happen during the Spring Classics, however, although you do not need to drink as much, you still need

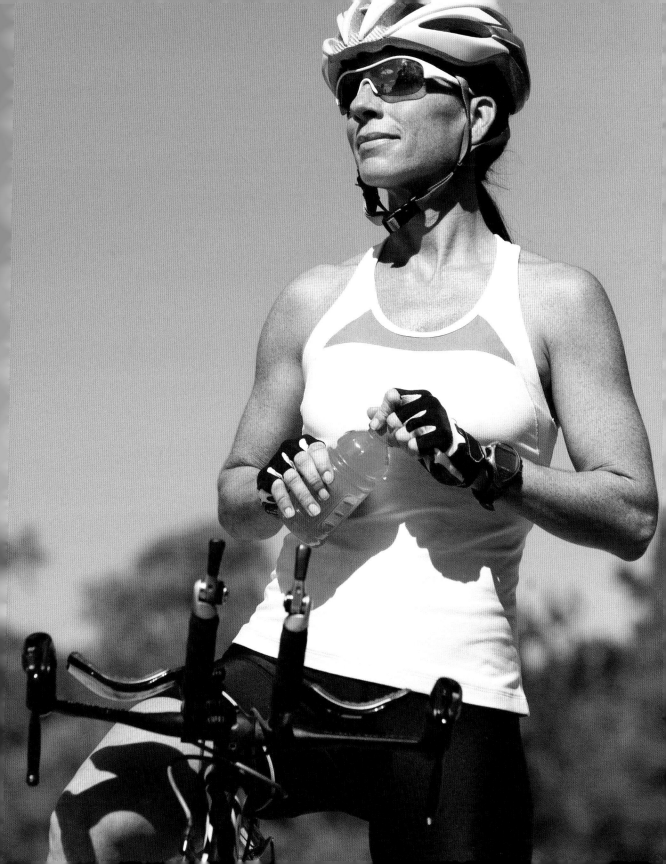

to drink. One way to ensure that you drink is to buy an insulated bottle and make a bottle of tea. The fact that the drink is warm encourages you to drink. My favourite is a fruit tea or herbal infusion or a green tea. You can squirt some honey or agave nectar in for some extra carbohydrates and sweetness. If you are not a good drinker during the winter, i.e. you go out for a three-hour ride and hardly touch your bottles, making tea can really encourage you to drink.

CAN I DRINK TOO MUCH?

You're more likely to adversely affect your performance and health by not drinking enough than by drinking too much. Our bodies are generally very good at getting rid of excess fluid and, if you drink too much, you'll just end up going to the toilet more. If you do take on too much water without adequate electrolytes, you can end up feeling bloated, nauseous and losing your desire to drink. In extreme and thankfully rare cases massive overconsumption of water can lead to a condition known as hyponatremia (low sodium concentrations). Cases of this have been seen in recent years at big, city-centre marathons, where runners, worried by constant reminders of the importance of staying hydrated, have drunk excessively before the event and taken plain water on at every single aid station. This has led to a few rare fatalities, but, for cyclists, as long as you balance your water and electrolyte consumption, it's not an issue.

CRAMP RUINED MY RIDE

Many riders who have suffered cramp during a long training ride, sportive or race, blame poor hydration and a lack of electrolyte intake for their painful demise, but recent studies have indicated that this isn't always the case. For such a common occurrence, it might surprise you to know that the exact reason for cramping is still unknown. Many people blame inadequate hydration or electrolyte levels and, although some studies have shown that consuming a 6 per cent carbohydrate sports drink can help prevent them, other studies have failed to back this up, including a recent study with Ironman triathletes, which found no link at all. Some studies of long-term sufferers of cramp have shown magnesium supplementation to be helpful.

Another factor attributed to causing cramps is a sudden increase in exercise intensity, so, if you suddenly ride harder or longer than you're used to, you can expect to cramp. However, exercise intensity can't be the only factor as it doesn't explain night cramps. Anecdotal evidence suggests that stretching can help to alleviate cramp and that regular stretching can help prevent cramp in muscles that are prone to it or that have previously been injured.

If cramp is a regular problem for you, either on the bike or off it, try the following:
- Review your pacing strategy. You're probably trying to ride too hard for your current fitness level. Follow a structured training plan and build up speed and distance gradually.

- Follow the hydration guidelines given in this chapter.

- Stretch regularly, paying particular attention to the muscle groups which normally cramp.

- Eat foods rich in magnesium and calcium, including leafy green vegetables, nuts, seeds and legumes.

PRO STORY: RACE-WINNING HYDRATION

The Grand Tours pose many nutritional challenges, but one of the biggest is managing hydration. Climatic conditions can vary massively from day to day and even during a single stage. It can be close to freezing on a high mountain pass, with the riders brushing their elbows on snow banks, but scorching hot on the flat valley roads once they've descended. It is therefore vitally important to constantly monitor hydration. I've already stated how important hydration is to recovery and it's often stated that the winners of Grand Tours are the riders who recover the best. It is testament to the professionalism of riders like Chris Froome and Sir Bradley Wiggins that, even under the unreliably testing and variable conditions of a Grand Tour, they show very little fluctuation of daily body weight and their overall hydration status. To achieve this though, on some days they would consume up to 10 l of fluid and, under the stress of racing, that takes an amazing amount of discipline.

If pro riders make hydration mistakes they can underperform. This often happens in the early part of the season during the Spring Classics. With narrow roads and cobbled sections, the racing is extremely stressful and you'll often get a hot day that catches everyone out. In a race some riders simply forget to drink so, if I know that a rider is susceptible to this, I'll make sure he has a reminder taped to his stem. If some pros need this, there's definitely no shame in you doing the same.

A few other hydration tips for the pros are:
- *If the temperature is over 25 °C (77 °F) aim to drink a bottle of water and a bottle of sports drink per hour on rides lasting over two hours.*

- *Have an insulated bottle. This will keep tea warm in the winter and drinks cold in the summer.*

- *On particularly hot days, fill a bottle about a third full and put it in the freezer overnight. Top up if necessary in the morning (remember, liquids expand when frozen). This will mean your drink stays cool for a good two hours.*

KNOWLEDGE TO TAKE AWAY

- **Cycling is unique** We've already discussed the unique demands of cycling, even for amateur riders, so don't try and apply studies of other sports or activities to your cycling. The hydration practices outlined in this chapter are tried and tested on the toughest cycling races on the planet.

- **Recovery** Along with the negative effects of dehydration on your performance while riding, it'll also negatively affect your body's ability to recover from a ride and impact on your next one. For a stage racer, hydration is key, but even if you're only training, it can be limiting your gains. Recovery is when the body adapts and becomes fitter. Compromise your recovery and the adaptations will be less and you'll also underperform in subsequent workouts.

- **Monitor** Check your hydration levels with daily weigh-ins and by using a urine colour chart (see page 228).

- **Sweat test** We're all individuals, so perform a sweat test to ascertain your hydration needs.

- **Try it in training** With all aspects of nutrition, as with bike set-up and kit, make sure you experiment with, and fine-tune, your hydration strategy in training. Find a sports drink that works, check that you can handle it in the volumes required by your target events and then stick to it.

- **Cramps** Hydration and electrolyte level may be a contributing factor to cramp, but it's more likely that you're just trying to ride too hard for your current ability.

HOMEMADE SPORTS DRINK 1

This first option makes a really light drink that's very easy on the stomach and is brilliant for hot days. If it's really hot, for a second bottle, freeze the pineapple juice and add the water and salt just before you head out.

Servings 1 (500 ml)
Calories per serving: 70 kcal
Carbohydrate per serving: 18 g
Fat per serving: 0.5 g
Protein per serving: 0.0 g
Sodium per serving: 440 mg

INGREDIENTS

250 ml pineapple juice
250 ml water
1 g LoSalt (or a
  low-sodium salt)

METHOD

1. Pour the pineapple juice, water and salt into a 500ml drinks bottle. Shake and enjoy.

HOMEMADE SPORTS DRINK 2

This second drink option delivers a higher amount of carbohydrate and can be more suitable for higher-intensity sessions where you need more of a boost. I use some apple juice in this, which provides the flavour, fructose and some electrolytes. I also use plain unflavoured maltodextrin, which can be easily bought from pharmacists and online retailers.

Servings 1 (500 ml)
Calories per serving:
    123 kcal
Carbohydrate per serving: 30 g
Fat per serving: 0 g
Protein per serving: 0 g
Sodium per serving: 0 g

INGREDIENTS
150 ml apple juice
20 g maltodextrin
350 ml water

METHOD
1. Put all of the ingredients into a drinks bottle and give it a shake.

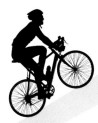

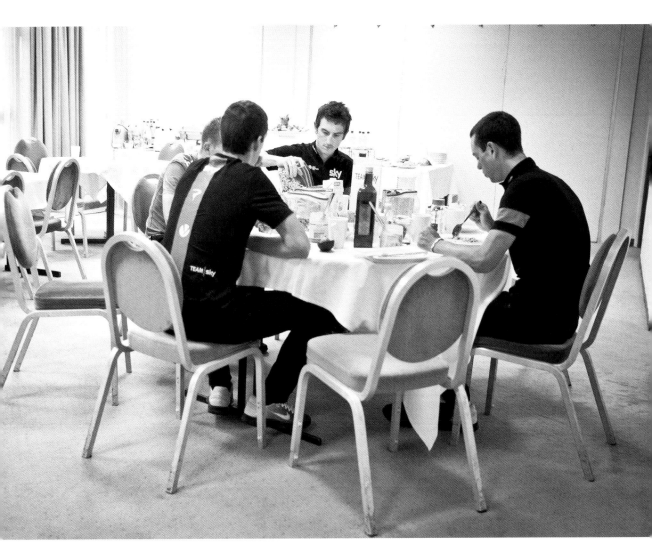

*Geraint Thomas and Richie Porte
of Team Sky eat breakfast at the
start of the seventh stage of the
2014 Tour de France*

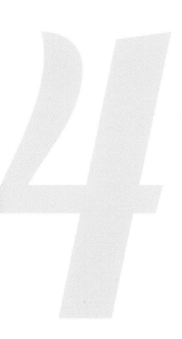

THE DAY BEFORE

What you eat on the day before a big event, race or training ride plays a massive role in how you'll perform the next day. You're laying the nutritional foundations for your efforts tomorrow and ensuring that the muscle glycogen stores that we talked about in Chapter 1 are fully topped up.

The past wisdom for preparing for endurance events was a convoluted routine of carbohydrate depletion followed by gorging yourself at pre-event pasta parties. Many amateur athletes even skipped the depletion phase and just saw it as an excuse for a massive pasta binge. This just isn't necessary or effective and will tend to result in unnecessary fat storage and a feeling of being bloated and sluggish the next day – hardly conducive to a good ride. Some riders make the opposite mistake. With a light day, complete rest or travel before an event, they cut back on their eating too much and manage to deplete their glycogen stores.

In the lead-up to a big ride, you will have tapered your training down and, because of this drop in workload, as long as you have been eating well, your muscle glycogen levels will have naturally risen to near full capacity. On the day before the ride, the emphasis should be on quality, not quantity, managing blood sugar levels, and making sure that along with the 'go nutrients' – protein, carbohydrates and fats – you're taking in the 'glow nutrients' – essential vitamins and minerals – too.

THE GLYCEMIC INDEX

In Chapter 1, we looked at the structure of carbohydrates and how this was related to their conversion to useable energy when consumed. For all carbohydrate-based foods, there is a scoring system, known as the Glycemic Index (GI), which indicates a food's effect on a person's blood sugar level. Pure glucose is used as the reference point and is given a score of 100. Although there are other factors that can affect how rapidly a food affects your blood sugar level, such as quantity consumed and whether the food is consumed with fat, protein or fibre, the Glycemic Index still provides a useful guide. As a general rule, high GI carbohydrates will give you a quick hit of energy whereas lower GI foods are more slow-burning.

Food	GI
Porridge (made with water and milk)	50
White rice	65
Potato, boiled	60
Sweet potato	40
Wholemeal bread	60

Sample GI ratings
(For a fuller list refer to the Carbohydrate Exchange List Ready Reckoner in the Appendix on page 229)

EATING THE DAY BEFORE

Start the day as you mean to go on; porridge made with milk or water is ideal. The oats provide slow-release energy and also essential B vitamins. If you're not keen on porridge, it's worth trying to acquire a taste for it as it really is great fuel for cyclists. You should also try to have some protein, so maybe also include an omelette or some yoghurt. This may seem like quite a big breakfast, especially as you're only likely to be doing a light spin today, but you don't want to make the mistake of undereating. Have a snack mid-morning; something like a banana is good just for keeping those carbohydrate levels topped up.

Your lunch should be simple and easily digestible. Opt for some grilled salmon or chicken for protein, and a very good choice for carbohydrates would be some sweet potato. Sweet potato, contrary to its name, has a lower Glycemic Index than regular potato so is perfect for getting those carbohydrates in but not pushing up the levels too rapidly. Don't forget to have some salad and vegetables too for those vital 'glow nutrients'.

The day before a big event you should also be taking steps to ensure you get a good night's sleep. At lunchtime you should stop consuming any caffeine. It's important you keep drinking though, so switch to fruit teas or herbal infusions and water to stay well hydrated. Again, as at mid-morning, you should have a snack mid-afternoon to keep your blood sugar level stable. Fruit and some nuts and seeds is the healthy choice, but with a big ride the following day, there's no harm in treating yourself to a slice of cake.

Your evening meal is all about ease of digestion. It's unbelievable that riders used to get up ridiculously early to have a steak for breakfast before a big race in the 1970s and 1980s. Not only did this cheat them of valuable hours of sleep, but it also meant they'd be riding with a large, undigested lump of meat in their gut. Avoid heavy proteins, such as red meat, the night before. They'll affect how you ride the next day and, because of the strain put on your digestive system, potentially disturb your sleep too; this is because if your body is working hard to digest food, your body temperature increases, which can keep you awake. Fish, chicken or turkey will be far easier for your stomach to cope with. Rice is probably the best carbohydrate source the night before a ride as it's so easy for your body to digest. You don't need a huge amount though; 200 g cooked weight is plenty. You might prefer to mix in some quinoa with your rice for variety and extra protein, and don't forget to include some vegetables and salad too. Avoid anything that's heavily spiced; plain, simple and digestible are your watchwords.

Before you go to bed, have some natural yoghurt as the casein in it is an excellent slow-release form of protein that will drip-feed into your system overnight. Finally, a drink of camomile tea with honey is the perfect pre-ride nightcap. The camomile will calm you and the fructose-rich honey will ensure that your liver glycogen

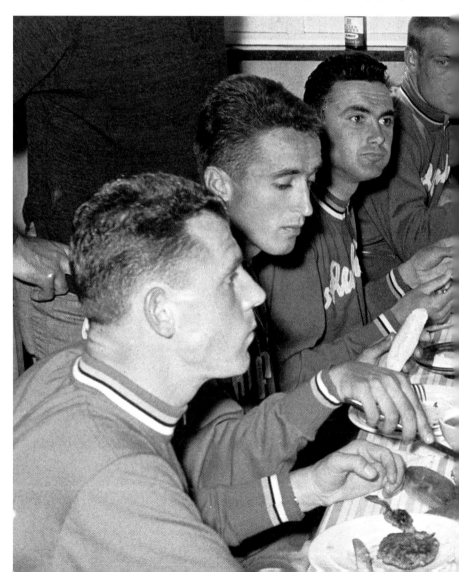

is topped up. Some people like to have a glass of wine to help them sleep, but, although it might help them get to sleep, even one glass will have a detrimental effect on sleep quality. Save having some wine or beer for celebrating after you've had a great ride.

TRAVEL TROUBLES

For many riders tackling a big event, the day before can mean having to travel and this can make eating well difficult. Preparation and organisation are key if you want to avoid being stuck with the unappealing and far-from-ideal fare offered by airports and motorway service stations. If you've made a big investment in terms

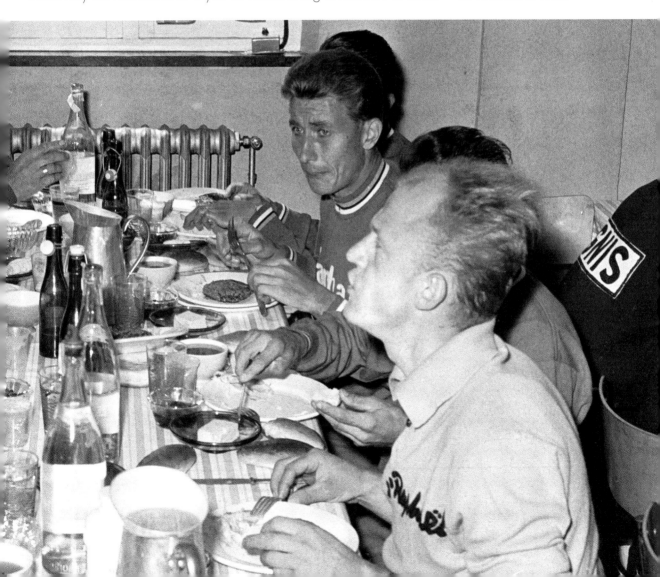

Teammates enjoy a meal during the 1962 Tour de France

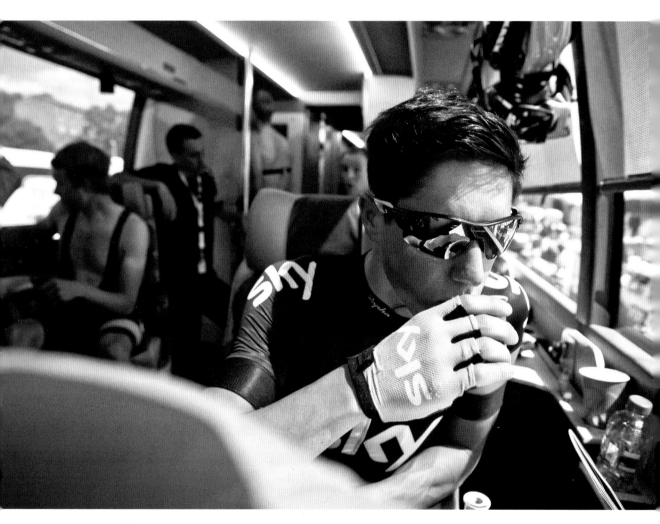

Peter Kennaugh of Team Sky has a
drink on the team bus after stage one
of the 2013 Tour de France

of training, entry fees, travel costs and accommodation expenses, I'd always advocate travelling 48 hours before your event and having a full day to get yourself sorted. It really takes the pressure off and means that your body, and potentially your bike, if you experience mechanical problems, will be better prepared. For a Grand Tour, pro riders will usually arrive three days before the start to ensure they're fully settled.

If you have no choice but to travel the day before, prepare for it. Pack some suitable food in Tupperware to cover the meals while you're travelling and don't forget healthy snacks too. On less high-profile stage races, the pros will often travel the day before. For the Tour of California, which Sir Bradley Wiggins won, he was working really hard on his weight and conditioning in the build-up and didn't want the long-haul flight to set him back, so he took his own food (rice, quinoa, homemade tomato sauce and chicken) to ensure he had what he needed.

We have all heard of and probably suffered from the condition known as jet leg. It occurs when we fly long-haul and our internal body clock struggles to keep up with the change in time zones. It's also usually compounded by uncomfortable seats, poor food while travelling, and dehydration due to cabin conditions or excessive alcohol consumption. Even shorter flights or long drives can lead to travel fatigue. This is where the extra pressure and stress of travel puts additional strain on the body. For example, catching an early flight really disrupts sleep and, without the sort of discipline shown by Wiggins and other pros, maintaining normal eating habits can be almost impossible. Try to plan the travel to be as less disruptive as possible to your normal routine and remember to keep well hydrated.

Although not nutritional advice, a final top travel tip that all the pros use, whether flying or on the bus, is to wear compression clothing. Either go for below-the-knee stockings or full-leg tights, but ensure they're medical grade and offer a graduated fit. They help blood return to your heart and stop your legs feeling bloated and heavy. Wear them for the whole journey and remove them once you arrive. There are many sports brands available, but if you are on a budget, the cheaper medical stockings are just as good. When I fly, even if it is a short flight, I always wear them and I feel much better for it.

Another common trap that riders fall into when travelling the day before an event is arriving late the night before and then spending hours wandering around looking for a restaurant. This means unnecessary time on your feet, a late meal and probably not the right food. Do some research beforehand (most hotels and restaurants have their menus online) and make a booking. If there does not look to be anything suitable, email your hotel and tell them what you require as you'll usually find most hotels will accommodate your requests.

DEALING WITH A NERVOUS STOMACH

If you're a rider who tends to suffer from a nervous stomach before a big ride, are usually forced to stop mid-ride to have a bowel movement or regularly suffer from gastrointestinal distress, you should try to eliminate these issues in training by finding a nutritional strategy that works for you. Ensure you've ticked all the boxes in the chapter on gut health (see page 25–39). Ease back on fibrous fruit and vegetables in the days leading up to your ride, but make sure you still get your 'glow nutrients' from vegetable juice or energised greens. Try following the low-residue diet (see pages 37–38) for the three days leading up to your event as this is very easy on your digestive system. Do remember to try it several times before training rides though as some riders do feel a bit flat having been on it. Avoid heavily spiced food and, even more so than other riders, be organised and prepared to ensure you get exactly the right food that works for you.

PRO STORY: FUELLING PARIS-ROUBAIX PART 1

Although they're one-day races, together the Spring Classics campaign is almost like a stage race. For many fans, it's all about Milan–San Remo, Tour of Flanders and Paris–Roubaix, but for pro riders, with all the semi-classics such as E3 Harelbeke, Gent–Wevelgem and Driedaagse De Panne, it's three weeks of almost back-to-back racing. In the short gaps between the races, the biggest issue is the riders getting bored and overeating. To prevent this, the nutritional routine is just kept really simple, following the same sort of plan as I've described earlier for before a big ride. On the days they're not racing, it's a balancing act of eating enough to keep their glycogen stores topped up, but not eating too much, ensuring their guts stay healthy and they're getting all of their key nutrients.

For Paris–Roubaix, the team will do a reconnaissance ride of the cobbled sections in the weeks leading up to the race. During the Classics, and the day before the race, the riders will have breakfast at their hotel and head out for a 60- to 90-minute ride. This is partly to keep their legs ticking over, but also to stop them getting bored. They'll then have a light lunch, usually finished up with natural yoghurt and fruit salad. It's then onto the bus for the drive to Compiègne.

As the team chef, I will have already travelled and got everything set up and ready for the riders. Meanwhile, on the bus, the riders will have some light snacks, such as energy bars, diluted fruit juice and some water. I'll have switched the coffee on the bus to decaf as it's vital for the riders to get a good night's sleep. The riders will arrive at the hotel at about four o'clock. Some will have a light massage and others will have a sauna; the sauna helps to get fluid out of the riders' legs that will have accumulated during the journey and it also helps them to relax. All of the riders will have worn compression clothing for the journey.

It's then back on the bus for a team briefing. I'll go through where feeds will be, though this is more for the support staff and, to be honest, it'll go over most of the riders' heads. The important thing is to ensure the idea of feeding is in their minds. Even the most experienced riders can get giddy on race day and forget to eat. They'll get to the finish and complain about bonking, but, when we look back, we'll find they just didn't eat. By constantly reminding them about feeding, even putting notes on their stems, it ensures that they're thinking about feeding.

We'll then all sit down to dinner between seven and eight o'clock. The aim is to have a relaxed atmosphere and for it to be business as usual. You'll feel far more relaxed, less likely to make stupid mistakes and will perform better. The riders will head off to bed at about nine o'clock, most with a cup of camomile tea. Try to learn from this approach for before your own big events. Find a routine that works and plan so that you can stick to it, even if you're away from home.

KNOWLEDGE TO TAKE AWAY

- **No need to load** Your body can only store a set amount of carbohydrate and, as you'll have probably been tapering, it's more than likely to be near to full. Guzzling huge plates of pasta will just make you feel bloated and sluggish.

- **Make sure you eat enough** With less activity, some riders lose their appetite or feel guilty about eating. Make sure you eat enough so that your glycogen levels are stocked up and your performance won't suffer.

- **Keep it simple** You really don't need to do anything special. Just eat simple and easily digestible food that you know works for you. Before an event is not the time to experiment.

- **Plan** Especially if you're travelling or staying away from home, plan to ensure that you get the right food when you need it. Don't waste all of those hours of training. If you fail to plan, you're planning to fail.

CHICKEN BREAST IN A SIMPLE TOMATO SAUCE ON A BED OF RICE AND QUINOA

Sir Bradley Wiggins' inflight meal of choice - need I say more?

Serves 1
Calories per serving:
   475 kcal
Carbohydrate per serving: 69 g
Fat per serving: 6 g
Protein per serving: 45 g

INGREDIENTS

150 g chicken breast, chopped
½ onion, finely chopped
1 garlic clove, peeled and finely chopped
400 g can chopped tomatoes (with mixed herbs, if preferred)
1 tsp olive oil
½ tsp paprika
35 g dry basmati rice
35 g dry quinoa
Salt and pepper, to taste

METHOD

1. Put the basmati rice and quinoa in a rice cooker and add double the weight of water. 70 g dry weight of rice and quinoa with 140 ml of water will create approximately 200 g of cooked weight. Switch on the rice cooker and let it do its job. Alterntatively, cook according to the packet's instructions.

2. Heat the olive oil and soften the onion and garlic, on a moderate heat.

3. Add the chopped chicken and cook together until the chicken is cooked through and no longer pink and the onion is golden.

4. Add the chopped tomatoes and simmer gently for about 10–15 minutes.

5. Season with paprika, salt and pepper to taste.

My top taste tip is to also add a few drops of Henderson's Relish, which is similar to Worcestershire sauce, and available online.

TURKEY BREAST STEAK WITH HOMEMADE SWEET POTATO WEDGES AND WILTED SPINACH

Containing quality, easily digestible protein, this is a high-protein meal with slow-release carbohydrates and 'glow nutrients' from the spinach. The turkey is also a really good source of beta-alanine.

Serves 1
Calories per serving:
 691 kcal
Carbohydrate per serving: 44 g
Fat per serving: 32 g
Protein per serving: 55 g

INGREDIENTS

200 g turkey breast, thinly sliced
1 medium sweet potato, cut into wedges
2 tsp olive oil
½ tsp paprika
100 g fresh spinach
1 tbsp pistachio nuts, chopped (optional)
½ garlic clove, peeled and chopped (optional)
Salt and pepper, to season

METHOD

1. Preheat your oven to 180 °C, Gas 4.

2. Clean the sweet potato, but don't peel it. Cut it into rough wedge shapes. Par boil for about 5 minutes. Drain the water and drizzle with half the olive oil, sprinkling on the paprika, salt and pepper. Transfer to a baking tray and roast for 20–30 minutes or until they feel soft when you prick them with a fork.

3. With about 15 minutes of the sweet potato cooking time left, season the turkey strips with salt and pepper and lightly drizzle with the remaining olive oil. Cook under a medium grill for about 4 minutes each side and remove from the heat.

4. While the turkey is resting, add the spinach to a pan with a splash of water. Cook on a moderate heat for about 5 minutes or until it's cooked down but is still firm. If liked, you can add the garlic for extra flavour, stirring it into the spinach, and top with the chopped pistachio nuts.

PISTACHIO PÂTÉ WITH HOMEMADE SWEET POTATO WEDGES AND WILTED SPINACH

Replacing the turkey for pistachio pâté still delivers all the key go and glow nutrients and is an ideal option to have cold when travelling.

Serves 6
Calories per serving:
    290 kcal
Carbohydrate per serving: 34 g
Fat per serving: 11 g
Protein per serving: 13 g

INGREDIENTS

100 g carrots, peeled and
    finely chopped
120 g celery, chopped
1 tsp cumin seeds
1 garlic clove, chopped
150 g leeks, trimmed and
    finely chopped
150 g dried split red lentils
1 tsp olive oil
100 g pistachio nuts, roasted
    and chopped
150 g quinoa
3 tbsp tomato purée (tomato
    paste)
300 ml water
½ tsp paprika
Salt and pepper, to season
(for sweet potato wedges and
    spinach, see page 70)

METHOD

1. Heat the olive oil and soften the garlic, leeks, carrots and celery with the cumin seed over a medium heat for about 5 minutes. Add the tomato puree.

2. Stir in the quinoa, red lentils and about two-thirds of the pistachios (save the rest to make a topping).

3. Add the water gradually until the fluid is absorbed and the lentils and quinoa are cooked. This will usually take about 15–20 minutes.

4. Season with paprika and add salt and pepper to taste. Put in a food processor and blend until smooth.

5. Spoon into a container and top with the remaining chopped pistachios. Serve warm or cold with sweet potato wedges and wilted spinach (see page 70).

Turkey breast steak (L)
and pistachio pâté (R) with
homemade sweet potato
wedges and wilted spinach

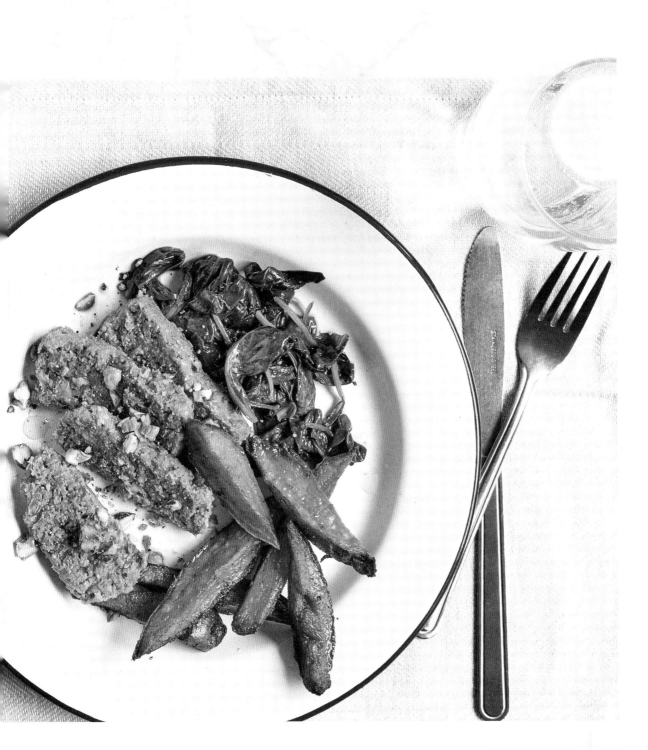

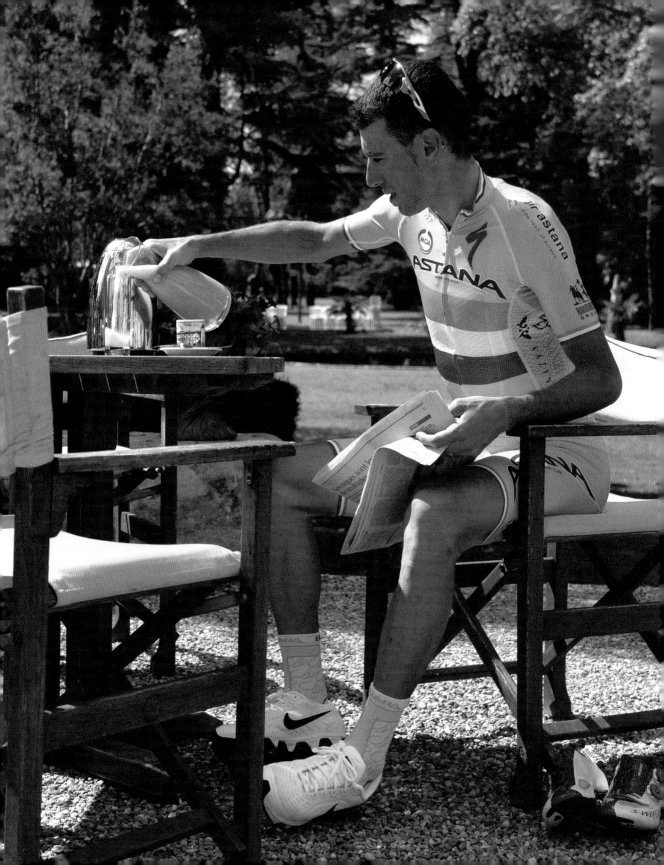

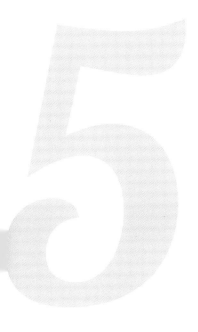

BREAKFAST

The commonly cited cliché is that breakfast is the most important meal of the day, but, assuming you've eaten and drunk well the day before a big event or ride, it's more a case of topping up your system and providing some fuel for the early kilometres of your ride. A good breakfast can also give you a bit of a psychological boost and comfort in the knowledge that you've got the fuel in your system to see you through your ride, so this shouldn't be underestimated.

When you wake up, your body is in a slightly depleted state. Even though you've been asleep, it has still been using energy. During the night, your brain is still active and glucose is needed to fuel this nocturnal activity. The glycogen stores in your liver are primarily there to maintain blood glucose levels and, as you sleep, you'll steadily tap these reserves. This is why I recommend having some camomile tea with honey before going to sleep; it'll help calm you down and give your liver's glycogen stores a bit of a boost. The priority in the morning then is to ensure that these stores are restocked. To do this, you don't need to have a massive breakfast, which is good news if you struggle to eat first thing in the morning, but equally, don't go too light as this could cause you to have doubts about whether you'll have enough energy in the tank. It's important not to overeat, but, for the sake of peace of mind, an extra serving of porridge or slice of toast isn't going to hurt.

WHAT TO EAT

Probably my number one breakfast choice for riders is porridge. It's warming, comforting and provides ideal slow-release carbohydrates. I'd always tend to pair it with an omelette or some yoghurt, either on top of the porridge or separately, to add some protein. Eggs are a brilliant choice to go with the porridge as their proteins and fats slow the digestion, absorption and release of energy from the carbohydrates. They effectively lower the Glycemic

Italy's Vincenzo Nibali pours himself a glass of orange juice during a rest day in the 2014 Tour de France

Index of the porridge oats and mean that you'll receive a steady trickle, rather than a deluge, of energy into your system.

It's interesting how things change in cycling. At Team Sky, when we started, many of the foreign riders had not had porridge before, but it soon became the staple of the team. Now it's funny that you see it on the breakfast table of nearly all pro teams. Finding porridge oats can be tricky in mainland Europe though and I used to buy it in bulk in the UK and take it over with me. (Just

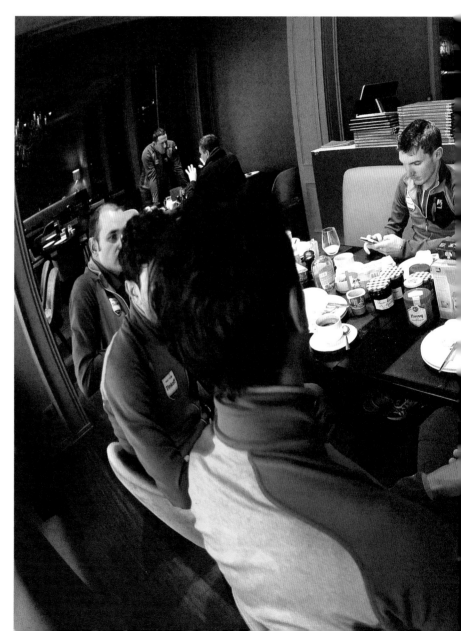

before the 2012 Tour, I had about 30 kg of porridge oats on the conveyer belt at my local supermarket and the checkout operator asked if I worked at a care home!) I also like a seed and Goji berry mix to add as a porridge topper. You should look to buy milled seeds so that you can easily digest and absorb the nutrients they contain; the whole seeds will tend to just pass straight through you.

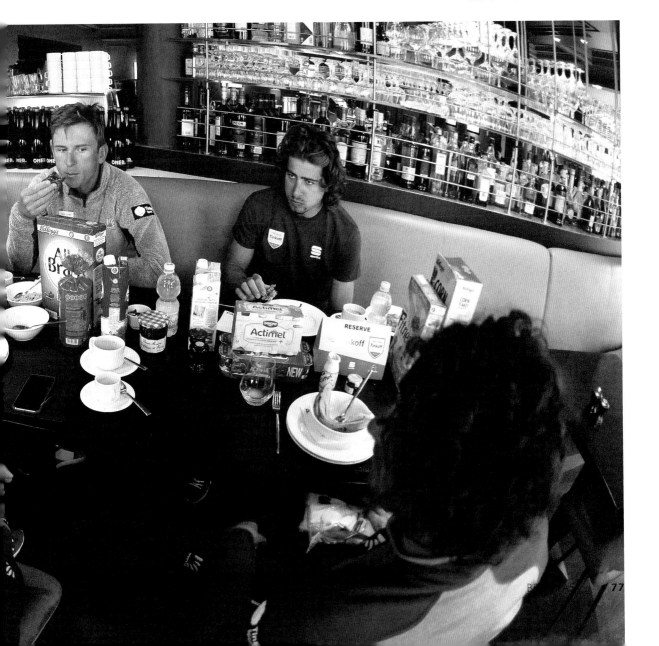

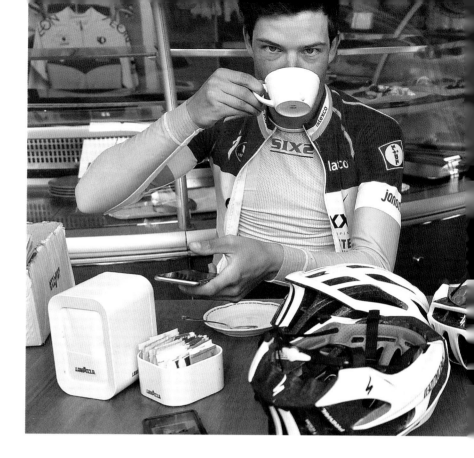

Gianluca Brambilla and Bob Jungels of Team Etixx–Quick-Step having a cappuccino on a rest day during the 2016 Giro d'Italia

Seeds are a great source of healthy fats, antioxidants and minerals. Pro cyclists tend to be a bit fearful of fat, but I've found that eggs are a great way of giving them the essential fats they need without causing them too much stress and anxiety. Some people do worry about the cholesterol in eggs, but in an active healthy person, there is little risk that it will contribute to raised blood cholesterol. Interestingly, there is some thought that the cholesterol in eggs may support testosterone levels. There is currently little scientific evidence to back this up, but cholesterol is a key component in the body's synthesis of testosterone.

If you tend to suffer from a sensitive stomach, a good option, which does sound a little strange for breakfast, can be basmati rice and an omelette. Make sure you choose basmati rice though as it has a lower Glycemic Index than regular white rice. All riders are different, so it's essential to experiment in training and find what

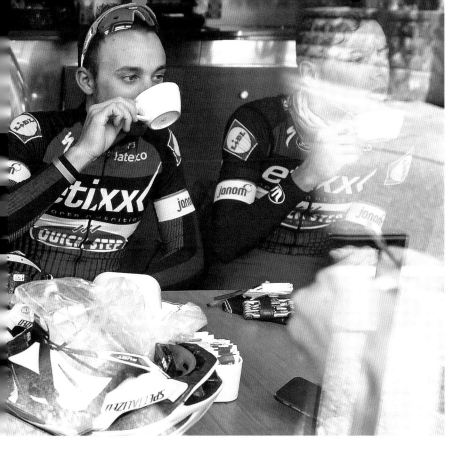

works best for you. I'd generally advise to stay clear of wholegrain and granary bread as it's very high in fibre and will tend to sit heavy in your stomach. Also, no matter how tempting it may be, the full English fried breakfast is never a good choice before a long ride.

Don't forget hydration. You should have been drinking well the day before so don't over-drink in the morning or you'll be forced into an early comfort break. Sip continuously and aim to consume about 500 ml water per hour in the lead-up to a ride. If you struggle to eat before a ride, you can use a sports drink to ensure you are getting enough carbohydrates.

For many cyclists, a coffee is an essential part of their pre-ride ritual. There's certainly no harm in including a couple of single-shot espressos with your breakfast, which will give you about 100 mg of caffeine. This will give you a bit of a lift and there's some evidence that it can also improve your ability to utilise fat as a fuel. If coffee is part of your daily routine, however, your body will be habituated to it and any potential performance benefits will be reduced. To get the most beneficial effects of coffee on your cycling for a key event, you may want to consider abstaining from it for seven days beforehand. This will allow any withdrawal symptoms, such as headaches and morning grumpiness, to pass and significantly reduces your level of habituation. A word of warning though, don't overdo the coffee pre-ride or you might find yourself having to take an extra trip or two to the bathroom!

HOW MUCH TO EAT

As a general rule of thumb, for a long ride you should be looking to consume 1 g of carbohydrate per kg of bodyweight for your breakfast. A 70 g serving of porridge will provide you with about 40 g of carbohydrates and, if you chop a banana into it, that'll give you another 20–40 g. For your omelette, you should be looking to use two or three medium eggs.

WHEN TO EAT

Ideally, you'd allow three to four hours between eating your breakfast and starting your event. Many riders get this wrong and end up starting their ride while still trying to digest their breakfast. In order for your digestive system to function effectively, it needs an adequate blood supply. When you start riding, much of that blood supply will be diverted to your working muscles, compromising digestion. This means that food can just sit in your stomach, leading you to feel bloated, nauseous, or, if you push hard, to even vomit. To allow three to four hours, can mean having to set an early alarm. Before the longest race in the professional calendar, Milan–San Remo, the riders will be up at 6 a.m. to have their breakfast. Often in training this is not possible, but it's not a problem because normally the first hour of a training ride would be steady and therefore you can carry on digesting your breakfast as you ride.

EARLY STARTS

Unfortunately, many sportives have start times as early as 7 a.m, and no matter how dedicated you are, setting an alarm for 3 a.m. or 4 a.m. isn't recommended. The loss of sleep and disruption to your daily rhythm will have too negative an effect on your ability to perform well. For really early starts, especially if you're away for an event and you'll be heading off before your hotel serves breakfast, a super-convenient option is a humble tin of rice pudding (remember, I used to feed my mum this in her 12-hour time trials) or rice cakes, which are a staple in the pro peloton. Rice pudding provides an almost perfect blend of carbohydrate, protein, fat and simple sugars and is incredibly easy to digest. You can probably get away with eating it as close to an hour to your roll-off time. If you know this is likely to be the case for your target event, you should try it in training. Set an alarm for
5.45 a.m., eat your rice pudding at 6 a.m. and be out on your bike by 7 a.m. Do this a few times in training to ensure it does work for you.

If you've overslept badly or are just running short of time, the only real option is to eat something really light, such as a banana or energy bar, start sipping on some energy drink, and go straight into your on-the-bike fuelling routine. This is far from ideal for long rides though as you'll be playing nutritional catch-up all day and you'll definitely be compromising your performance or training benefits. Remember to set an extra alarm next time!

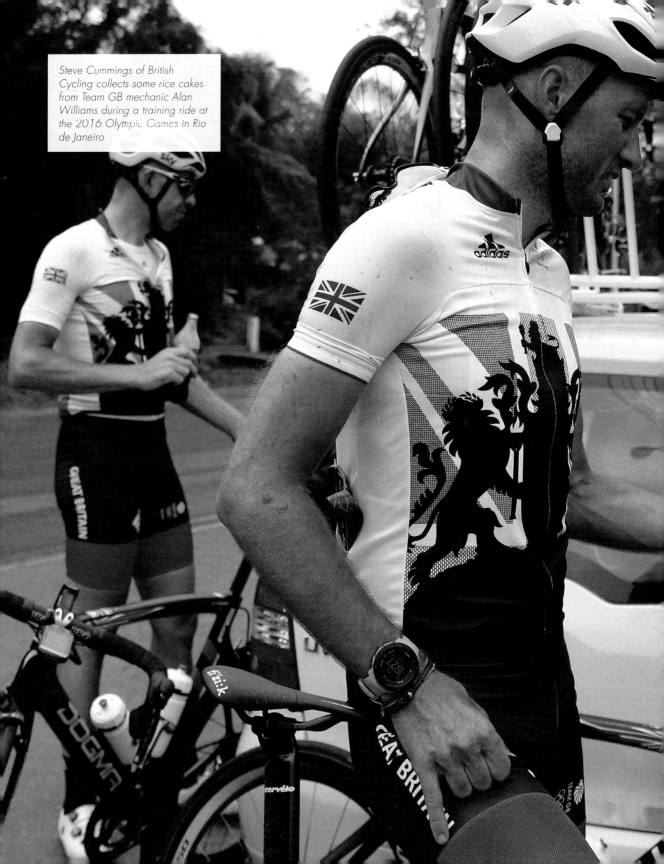

Steve Cummings of British Cycling collects some rice cakes from Team GB mechanic Alan Williams during a training ride at the 2016 Olympic Games in Rio de Janeiro

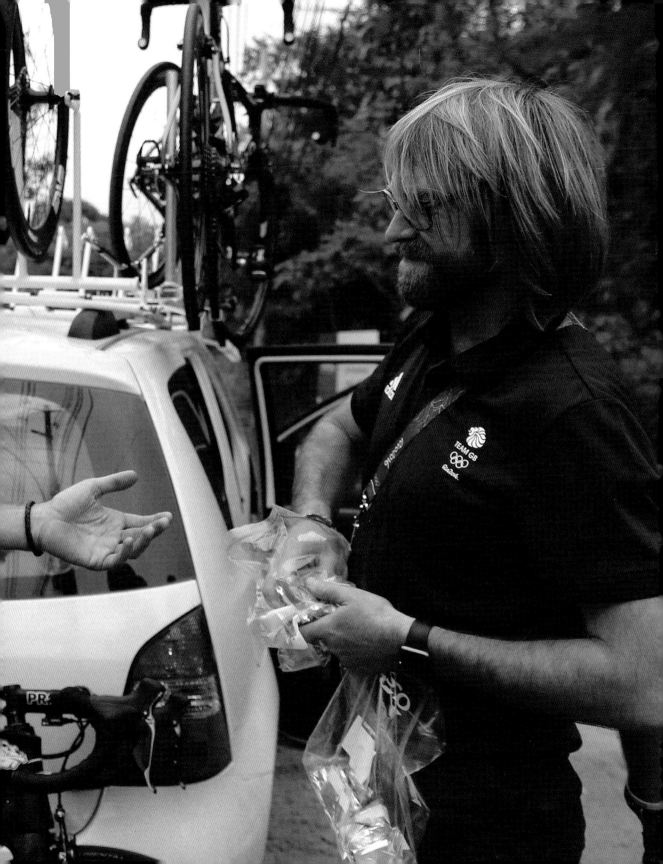

Start of the ride

How hard you're riding and your ability to fuel well on the bike are intrinsically linked and we'll explore this key relationship more in the next chapter. However, the intensity at which you start off your ride can also have a significant bearing on your breakfast. If it's a steady-paced training ride, club run or a sportive with a relatively flat start, you'll be able to ease into the ride and could probably get away with having your breakfast nearer to your start time.

As you're not riding hard, your muscles require less blood flow and therefore a decent supply will still be servicing your digestive system. However, if you know that a ride will be hard from the off, try to allow the full three to four hours.

The final few hours

With at least a few hours between your breakfast and starting your ride, you'll want to have a couple of light snacks. These are more for comfort and reassurance, but will also contribute to the opening kilometres of your ride. Opt for an energy bar, rice cakes or a banana and don't forget to keep sipping on some fluid.

PRO STORY: FUELLING PARIS-ROUBAIX PART 2

When we left the riders, they'd just had their camomile tea and were drifting off to sleep. However, for the support staff, the chef, mechanics and soigneurs, the day is far from over. Bikes have to be prepared, bottles and musettes made up and prep work for tomorrow's breakfast done. All the riders have to worry about in the morning is getting down for breakfast at 6.30 a.m., having their cases ready for pick-up at 7.30 a.m. and being on the bus for 8.00 a.m. Although you won't have an army of support staff for your events, you should do everything you can to minimise stress and uncertainty during those final 48 to 72 hours.

Breakfast is normally quite a subdued and professional affair. It's early and the riders and staff are focusing on one of the most important days of the year. Exactly what's eaten will vary from rider to rider, but it'll meet the basic principles of slow-release carbohydrates and protein. By the time the riders are having their breakfast, the mechanics and soigneurs, who'll have already been up for hours, will already have all the bikes, spares and supplies for the day loaded up and ready to go.

Once on the bus, the riders will have a final race briefing. The directeur sportif will have decided where he wants 'zone hoppers' placed with spare wheels, gels and bottles. These are fairly unique to the cobbled classics, where the rough and narrow roads mean that getting a team car to a rider can be almost impossible. There's a real community feel to these races and the zone hoppers are often long-time volunteers. The riders will be made aware of their locations and any changes to the team tactics, and, although they won't be given specific nutritional advice, we'll make sure that fuelling and hydration are in their minds. During the bus ride, the riders will snack on an energy bar, rice cake and some might have an extra cup of coffee.

Once the riders are on the bus to the start, the support team will decamp to the finish hotel. After Paris–Roubaix, the team chef might have a night off as there's usually a bit of a party to celebrate the end of the cobbled classics. However, although the riders can let their hair down a bit and maybe have a beer, many will be heading straight down to the Ardennes for more tough racing.

KNOWLEDGE TO TAKE AWAY

- **Topping up** If you've fuelled and hydrated well the day before, you don't need to eat a huge amount for breakfast, but for your own peace of mind, eat enough so you feel confident.

- **Carbs and protein** A balanced pre-ride breakfast should contain carbohydrates and protein. If you suffer from a nervous stomach, basmati rice and an omelette is ideal.

- **Allow time** For optimum performance, you should allow three to four hours between having your breakfast and starting your ride. There are solutions if an early start doesn't make this an option, but try to stick to it whenever possible.

- **Try it in training** Work through your exact pre-ride routine, especially if it's an unusually early start time, at least a few times before an important event.

- **Minimise stress** The pros only have to worry about getting up, eating breakfast and getting on the bus. You might not be able to achieve quite this ideal, but a bit of planning can avoid a lot of rushing around, panic and stress on the morning of a ride.

PERFECT PORRIDGE

··

This recipe can be made with water or milk. For the pros, we tend to use water. I like to use small organic oats with this recipe.

Serves 1
Calories per serving:
   198 kcal
Carbohydrate per serving: 36 g
Fat per serving: 4 g
Protein per serving: 6 g

INGREDIENTS

150 g porridge oats
½ apple, pear or banana, chopped
Pinch of cinnamon
100 ml water

METHOD 1

1. Put all the ingredients in a microwave-proof container, stir and cook in microwave on medium for two minutes.

2. Stir again and cook for a further minute.

3. Leave to stand for a minute and then give it a final stir.

If you like thick porridge, add less water. If you like it runny, add a little more water.

METHOD 2

1. If you do not want to use a microwave, cook in a heavy-based pan. Warm the water, add the fruit and let it simmer for 5 minutes until the fruit softens.

2. Gradually add the oats and a pinch of cinnamon while stirring. Simmer over a very low heat for 3–4 minutes. You will probably need to add a little more water.

OMELETTE

If there's one thing that a chef on a pro cycling team has to be able to do, it's to turn out delicious soft and fluffy omelettes. An omelette should be soft, fluffy, and definitely not rubbery. Many people overcook omelettes, which can denature the proteins, altering their chemical structure and making them hard to digest.

Serves 1
Calories per serving:
   221 kcal
Carbohydrate per serving: 0 g
Fat per serving: 19.4 g
Protein per serving: 22 g

INGREDIENTS
3 medium eggs (I use free range)
1 tsp olive oil
Salt and pepper, to taste
Optional:
A few cherry tomatoes, halved
A few mushrooms, halved
Chives, finely chopped, to sprinkle

METHOD

1. Crack the eggs into a bowl with some salt and pepper to taste and whisk well.

2. Warm a non-stick skillet or pan for a few minutes on a gentle heat and cover the base with olive oil. The oil will heat quickly and is ready when it becomes runny; if it is smoking, it is too hot. To double-check the heat, drop a small amount of egg into the pan and it should quickly cook, but not fizzle.

3. Add the omelette mixture to the pan. Stir it gently until it begins to set. Then just use a spatula to lift it around the sides to ensure it doesn't stick.

4. After a couple of minutes it should be firm enough to fold. Give it a little squeeze with the spatula: if it's a bit runny, it needs a bit more cooking. Serve with fried tomatoes or mushrooms, if desired, and a sprinkle of chopped chives.

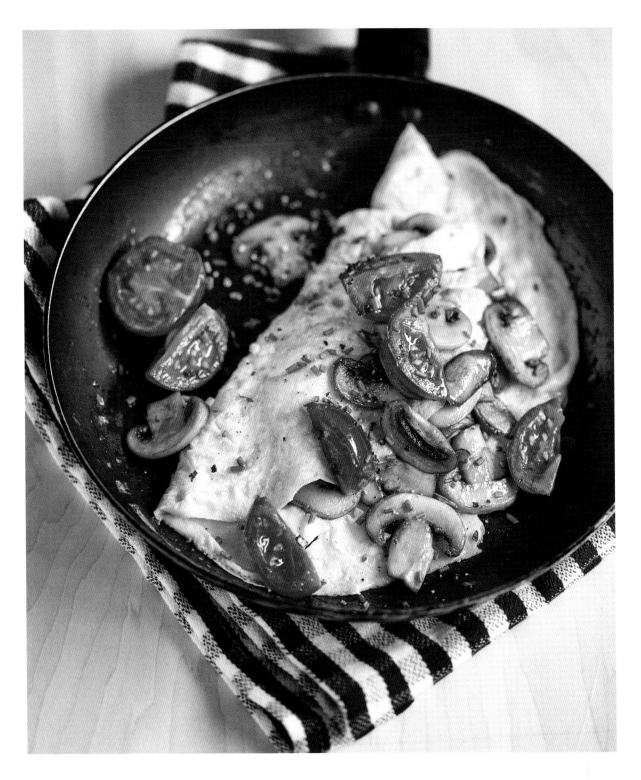

QUINOA AND COCONUT MILK PORRIDGE

A higher-protein alternative to regular porridge.

Serves 1
Calories per serving:
  482 kcal
Carbohydrate per serving:
  84 g
Fat per serving: 8 g
Protein per serving: 14 g

INGREDIENTS
30 g quinoa flakes
150 ml unsweetened
  coconut milk
150 ml water
Pinch of cinnamon
½ banana, chopped
Pinch of desiccated
  coconut (optional)

METHOD

1. Put the quinoa flakes in a pan, cover with the water and bring to the boil.

2. Reduce the heat and simmer for 10–15 minutes.

3. Stir in the coconut milk, cinnamon and chopped banana and cook for a further 5 minutes until creamy. Sprinkle with cinnamon and dessicated coconut, if liked.

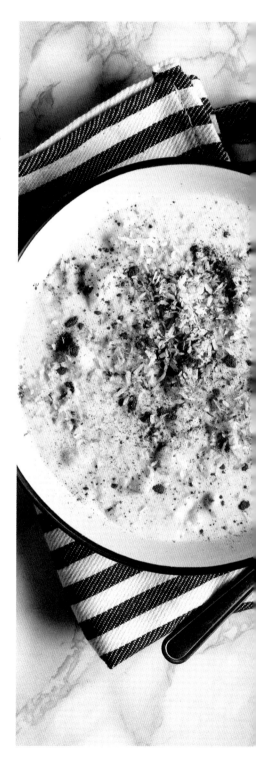

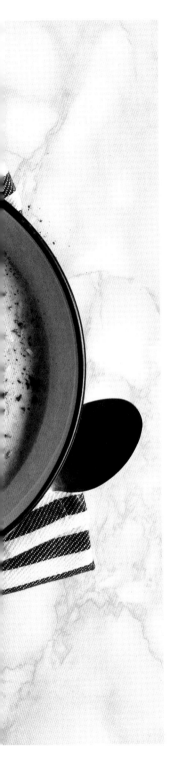

CHOCOLATE, SEED, NUT AND BERRY PORRIDGE TOPPING

A delicious way to add healthy fats, antioxidants and minerals to your porridge. This seldom lasts that long in my house. A pro team will get through this mix in two breakfasts!

Servings 10–20
   (1 serving is 2 tbsp
   or 30 g)
Calories per serving:
   144 kcal
Carbohydrate per serving:
   9 g
Fat per serving: 9.6 g
Protein per serving: 5 g

INGREDIENTS
50 g cocoa nibs
50 g dried Goji berries
50 g linseeds or
   flaxseeds, whole
50 g pistachio nuts,
   roasted and unsalted

METHOD

1. Put all of the ingredients in a blender, and blend on full speed for about 10 seconds. For the right texture, the nut and berry bits should be no more than a couple of millimetres big. It's important that the seeds are well-milled, otherwise they pass straight through you.

2. Put the mix in an airtight container. It will keep in the fridge for up to 10 days.

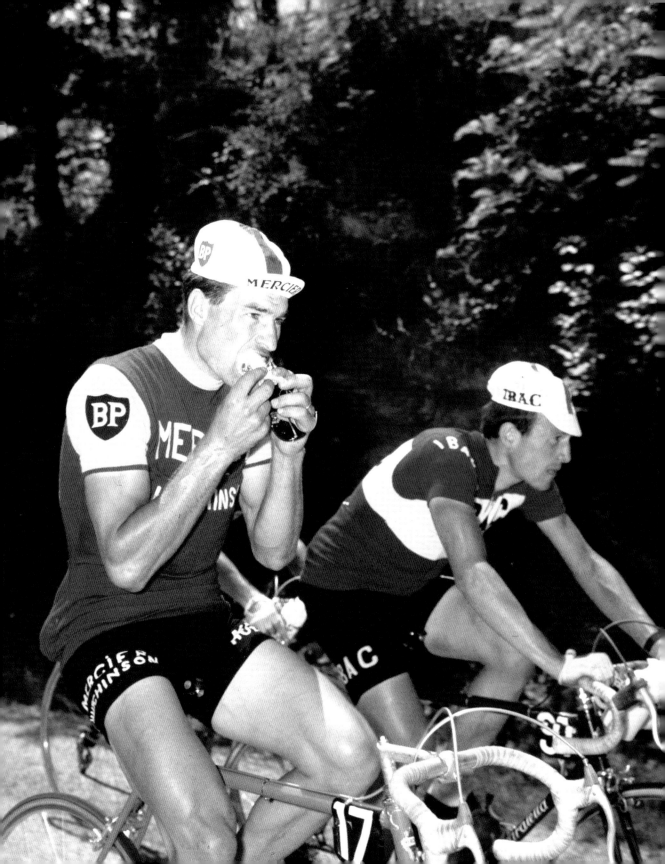

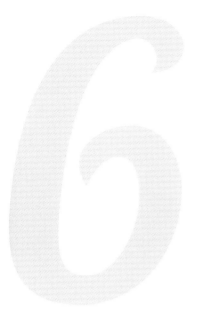

EATING ON THE BIKE

As we've previously discussed, one of the aspects of cycling that makes it a unique sport is that you can easily eat and drink while doing it. It's this fact that makes a 24-hour time trial, a three-week Grand Tour or extreme endurance events, such as the Race Across America, possible. You can replace the carbohydrates that you're burning so, in conjunction with drawing on your body's fat reserves, incredible feats of cycling endurance are possible. However, exactly what to eat, when and how much, will be determined by your individual digestive system and the type of ride you're undertaking.

IMPORTANCE OF INTENSITY

How hard you're riding, the amount of fuel you'll need and what you're able to tolerate are intrinsically linked. If you've ever suffered from digestive problems on a ride, such as ending up feeling bloated or nauseous and seemingly unable to get energy from the food you're putting in, it's more than likely that you were simply riding too hard for your ability. During hard exercise, blood is diverted from the digestive system (splenic blood system) to the peripheral working muscles. So, even though you can eat and drink on the bike, you have to be thoughtful about what you eat and how hard you ride. As the intensity of your riding increases, the food you consume has to become more easily digestible. You might just get away with pie and chips at the café stop on a very gentle club run, but try the same for a chain gang and the results wouldn't be pretty! For this reason, along with following a structured training plan, you should be aware of how to pace your riding and monitor intensity. Heart rate monitors provide an affordable and effective option for many riders, but power meters, now that prices are starting to really drop, should be high on the wish list for any semi-serious cyclist.

Power meters have revolutionised how cyclists train and

Raymond Poulidor eats on his bike during the 1963 Tour de France race. They have been around for about 20 years and are now universally used by top cyclists. An analogy of how important they've become is, in the view of top cycling coaches, that a cyclist training on the bike without a power meter would be like an athlete training in the gym with all the kilogram markings on the plates taped over. Prices are really starting to drop due to patents expiring and more manufacturers entering the market, and a number of manufacturers are now offering single-sided units. These measure power from one pedal or crank arm and then extrapolate the data for both sides to obtain total power. Unless you have major pedal stroke imbalances, their accuracy is totally acceptable and they are very affordable. I would expect over the next few years that more and more amateur riders will convert to using power meters and reap the benefits of it.

Power meters are not without their critics; some say they remove the spontaneity from racing and reduce the riders to robots, but you have to remember that a power meter doesn't turn the pedals for you! What they do give is an amazing and instantaneous insight into how hard a cyclist is riding and a degree of accuracy for training and racing that just simply didn't exist previously. This means that riders can train and perform better, but also that the training stress that they're putting on their bodies can be accurately measured, resulting in smarter and healthier training practices. From a nutritional perspective, we're only just beginning to scratch the surface of what power meters can do. Certainly, as they make pacing more accurate, riding at an intensity that allows you to fuel is definitely easier. They also offer a more accurate measure of the calories burned during a ride than from heart rate monitoring. However, this figure, which won't take into account a rider's fitness or efficiency and is solely based on physical work done, should still only be taken as an estimate. As we develop our understanding of power data and as analytical software is improved and integrated with existing knowledge of sports science and physiology, the possibilities are extremely exciting. It won't be long until we're able to see in real time how many and how quickly a rider is burning calories and also what percentage of those calories are from carbohydrates and what are from fats. Riders will effectively have a fuel gauge like a car and my job as a nutritionist will be a whole lot easier!

If you're not currently riding using a heart rate monitor, or ideally a power meter, it should be a priority to test regularly (every six to eight weeks) for your Functional Threshold Heart Rate (FTHR) or Functional Threshold Power (this represents the effort that you can sustain for about 45–60 minutes at a constant intensity) and use this to set personalised training zones. Don't rely on age-based formulae or automatic zone calculation functions on heart rate monitors or bike computers. They're too generic and will give you widely inaccurate zones. There are a number of testing protocols you can follow, but I recommend British Cycling's and their zone calculator, which can be easily found on their website: (www.britishcycling.org.uk).

When I talk about heart rate and power zones in this book, these are the percentage bands of FTHR and FTP that I'm referring to:

	Definition	Percentage of FTHR (heart rate)	Percentage of FTP (power)
Zone 1	Active recovery	< 68%	<55%
Zone 2	Endurance	68–83%	55–76%
Zone 3	Tempo	83–93%	76–90%
Zone 4	Threshold	93–105%	90–105%
Zone 5	VO_2 max	105–120%	105–120%
Zone 6	Anaerobic capacity	n/a	120–150%

Power zones and percentage bands of Functional Threshold Heart Rate (FTHR) and Functional Threshold Power (FTP)

CREATING A BETTER GEL

Gels are an accepted and convenient way to fuel harder efforts on the bike. However, many riders struggle to digest them, especially if they're having to use them in large numbers over the course of a long ride. In the build-up to the London 2012 Olympic Road Race, we found that most of the GB riders were OK taking two to four gels regularly, but were struggling to stomach any more. This created a problem as, during the race, we calculated that they'd need 10+ gels. We came up with the idea of using natural undiluted fruit juice with added maltodextrin to make a far more liquid gel and fed these to the riders in zip-tie bags. They worked, we got good feedback and so we got some properly made up for the race. A major factor in the success of these gels was the concept of multi-substrate fuelling. For some time now, we have known that absorption from the gut into the body can be one of the limiting factors for energy delivery. Including some fructose (fruit sugar) in the gel can provide an additional delivery pathway. Glucose uses one channel in the gut and fructose another, so if the glucose pathway is 'clogged' up, the fructose can act as an additional channel for energy absorption. The beauty of the fruit juice gels is that fruit juice naturally contains fructose. You have to be careful not to overdo the fructose though, as, in excess, it can cause stomach problems. However, in a typical gel delivering 20 g of carbohydrate, if 5 g is provided by fructose, this shouldn't be a problem.

I'm really proud of having been part of the development of these type of gels, with a higher water content, natural ingredients and multi-substrates, and they are now widely available. If you tend to struggle with stomaching other gels, you should definitely try them.

NOT ALL RIDES ARE FUELLED THE SAME

You'll often read books or magazine articles that tell you to eat X amount of carbohydrate per hour and pretty much leave it at that. However, in the same way that more riders are taking a more analytical and scientific approach to their training, you should be doing the same with your nutrition. It's important to look at the demands of each particular ride, race or workout, regarding intensity and duration, and to plan your nutritional strategy accordingly. This will ensure that you perform optimally during that ride and maximise the training gains you get from it. We'll look at fuelling guidelines for a number of typical sessions here, but, in Chapter 11, more riding and racing scenarios, such as an evening 10-mile time trial, criterium or cyclocross race, are covered with detailed nutritional timelines.

The Sunday club run and steady-paced endurance ride

Make sure you get up in time so that you can have a decent breakfast. This will ensure that all your energy stores are well-stocked. The majority of a typical club run will be ridden at a social pace in Zones 1 and 2 (see table on page 95), but there will always be a few spikes as you sprint for town or village signs, or hit a particular climb. Even without these higher-intensity efforts, because of the large amount of muscle mass that even riding at relatively low intensities recruits, you'll be starting to chip away at your carbohydrate reserves. After about 60 minutes without food you'll still have carbohydrate stores left in your body, but your blood glucose level will be starting to drop. For this reason, after about 45 minutes of riding, look to take on 20 g of carbohydrates. This could be in the form of a sports drink, a rice cake, a banana, a small panini or about half of a typical energy bar. You could use a gel, but at this sort of ride intensity, you're better off with solid food. If you imagine the food you eat as being like the fuel for a fire, then a gel is like a fire lighter. It burns fast and hot, but doesn't

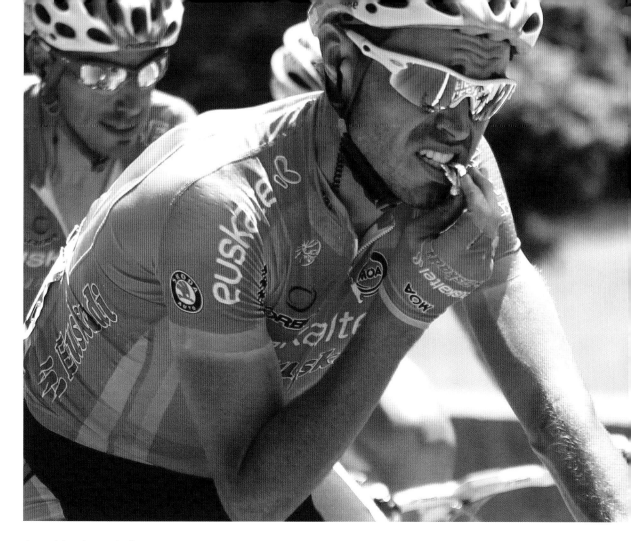

Samuel Sanchez and Alberto Contador consume energy gels during the 2010 Tour de France

last long. Great if you need a quick energy boost or are suffering from a bit of a bonk, but not so good for long-steady-paced efforts. For this type of ride, solid food burns a bit like a lump of coal. It'll give out the same amount of energy, but much slower. You should aim to take on another 20 g of carbohydrate every 30–45 minutes for the remainder of the ride.

If your club ride tends to get a bit competitive during the run in to the café stop, this can be the time to use a gel. Take it before the pace starts to ramp up and it'll give you a bit of a boost. Don't forget to factor the café stop into your nutritional plan for the ride. If you've been regularly taking on fuel during the ride before hitting

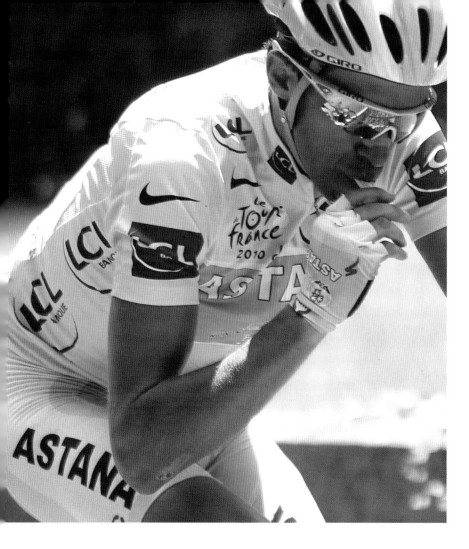

the café, you won't get there feeling ravenous and needing to devour half the menu. Some beans or scrambled eggs on toast or a scone will probably be plenty. Don't be the rider who doesn't eat a thing on his bike, tucks into a full English fry-up at the café and is then moaning about feeling bloated and uncomfortable for the rest of the ride!

Sportives

With a sportive, or a training ride in preparation for one, you're likely to be out riding for three to six hours. Again, eat well the day before and follow my breakfast advice to ensure you've laid down some solid nutritional foundations. Although you're likely to be riding in Zones 1 and 2 on the flats, there will be more intensity on the climbs, where you'll be pushing through Zone 3 and up into Zone 4.

Many sportives also tend to start off fast and, unless you're super-disciplined about your pacing plan, it's hard not to get sucked into the excitement of the event and overcook the first 30–40 minutes. Be ready for this and prepared to eat a bit more and a bit earlier than on steady paced training rides; maybe have your first feed after 20 minutes. If you can resist joining in the mad dash away from the line and ease yourself into the ride, this is definitely preferable and you'll almost definitely end up passing those riders who shot off later on. As a general plan, stick to the 20–30 g of carbohydrate every 30–45 minutes, but you have to do this like clockwork throughout the ride. It's worth setting a reminder on your bike computer, watch or taping a note to your stem. Even pro riders do this because, in the excitement of a race, they'll forget to eat. It's really unpleasant and difficult to dig yourself out of a blood sugar crash so avoid it by eating little, early and often throughout the ride.

Do some research on the route because, in addition to your regular feeds, if there are some significant climbs, it can be a good idea to have a gel five minutes before hitting its base. Even if you've taken on some regular food fairly recently, a gel can still give you a much-needed boost for the higher-intensity climbing effort. Just the act of having a sugary substance in your mouth will give you an initial lift and then, as you climb, the fast-release carbohydrates will kick in. In the mouth are receptors that detect the 'sweet' taste from the gel and send a signal to the brain that there is carbohydrate on its way. This in itself can give a performance boost before the energy has even hit the bloodstream. Depending on the length of the climb, you might also want to take a feed as you go over the top. You won't be working hard as you descend and this makes it far easier for your body to digest and absorb food. Watch any pro race in the mountains and you'll see the riders fuelling up in this way as they crest a major climb.

On most sportives you'll have a number of feed stations, but my advice is to try and not rely on them, but be as independent about your nutrition as possible. All it takes is for the event organiser's logistics to be slightly out and you could be rolling into a feed station with nothing but banana skins left. Even for a four- to six-hour ride, it's not too difficult to carry all the food you'll need and that way you know you won't miss out. If you do decide to use the feed stations, do some research before the event about where they're situated and what they're offering. Make sure you try the products that'll be used in training to check that you can tolerate them. I'd still recommend carrying a stash of your own gels for climbs, in case you have a sugar crash or if a feed station lets you down.

What you won't be able to carry is enough liquid for the ride and you will be reliant on feed stations to refill your bottles. Again, check which sports drink they're using and try it in training. Alternatively, bag up some of your own tried-and-tested sports drink powder in bidon portions and make this up with plain water from the feed stations.

Finally, maintain your nutritional discipline right through to the end of the event. It's a really common mistake for riders to think they only have 5–10 km remaining and to skip a scheduled feed. All it takes is a puncture, an unexpected climb or for the event organiser's distances to be a bit out and you'll be limping to the finish.

Evening chain-gang

Many riders will be doing this type of quality session in the evening. To make sure you're prepared, you'll need to work back from your start time and ensure you have a suitable snack three hours beforehand. This doesn't need to be huge if you've been eating well during the day and could be a sandwich, a baked potato, some pasta or even good old rice pudding. I would also suggest a little top-up of a banana about one hour before.

Including riding there and home, you'll probably be out for about two hours in a chain-gang session, which will include sustained Zone 3 and 4 efforts and maybe even higher when you hit the front. During your 30-minute warm-up ride to the start of the chain-gang, with about 10–15 minutes left, take on a snack, such as a banana, rice cake or energy bar. During the hour-long chain-gang effort, assuming you don't get dropped, you should be aiming to have a couple of feeds that'll deliver 40–60 g of carbohydrate. Again, bananas and rice cakes can work, but you might struggle to eat and digest denser energy bars. However, during this sort of ride the technical nature of riding through and off at speed can make eating solid food really tricky. This is where either using a carbohydrate sports drink or gels really comes into its own. It's funny how many riders finish a chain-gang with food still in their jersey pockets because they just haven't had the chance to eat it and then end up limping home, deep in a blood-sugar low. During your cool-down spin home, if you've got more hard training the next day, you can start your recovery by sipping on a recovery drink as you ride. Just take a sachet of your preferred recovery drink with you and mix it up with a second bottle of water. If you're not training the next day, this isn't so important, but still keep sipping and make sure you eat fairly soon after you get home.

Structured intervals within a ride

If you're working with a coach or following a training plan, you're likely to have sessions where you'll perform high-intensity intervals within a ride. This type of session is typically 90 minutes to three hours in duration, but for pro riders, it's not uncommon for these rides to be up to five hours.

As ever, make sure you eat well in the lead up to your session. Whether it's breakfast, lunch or an afternoon snack, work back and allow that three to four hours of digestion time. This is especially important for hard efforts as, during them, blood flow to your digestive system will be severely limited and you don't want food sitting in your stomach.

Typically, you'll perform an extended warm-up, your main interval set and then finish with a fairly long cool-down. You should be looking to perform your hardest efforts towards the front end of the ride when you're feeling most fresh. Fuel the warm-up section of the ride in the same way as a steady paced endurance ride. Stick a lump of coal on – solid food such as a banana, rice cake or half an energy bar, totalling about 20 g of carbohydrate – and repeat every 30–45 minutes. Your intervals will probably total 20–40 minutes of quality work with rest periods in between and you should break this chunk of the ride into thirds. Take one gel a third of the way through and a second, ideally caffeinated, two-thirds in. This is when you're likely to be really suffering, your blood sugar levels will be dropping and you'll need that boost.

As well as placing a big energy demand on your body, high-intensity efforts are metabolically very damaging too and result in large amounts of muscle damage. This is no bad thing as it's this damage which provides a training stimulus, and as it repairs, your body becomes stronger. Remember, your fitness increases when you are recovering, not training, so rest and recovery are critical. Optimal nutrition is one of the key drivers in this adaptation to exercise. A top coach once told me that he had never met an over-trained rider, just under-recovered. However, you have to provide it with the correct nutrients to facilitate this repair and recovery. We'll discuss the details of recovery in the next chapter, but in the same way as when you're riding home from a chain-gang, starting your recovery by sipping on a protein-rich recovery drink during the cool-down phase of your ride is optimal.

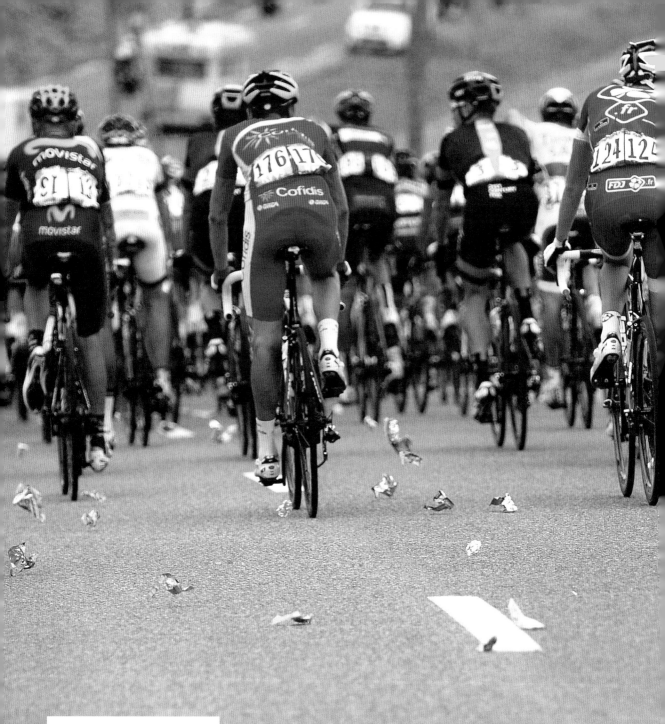

The peloton leaves the feed zone during the 15th stage of the 2014 Tour de France

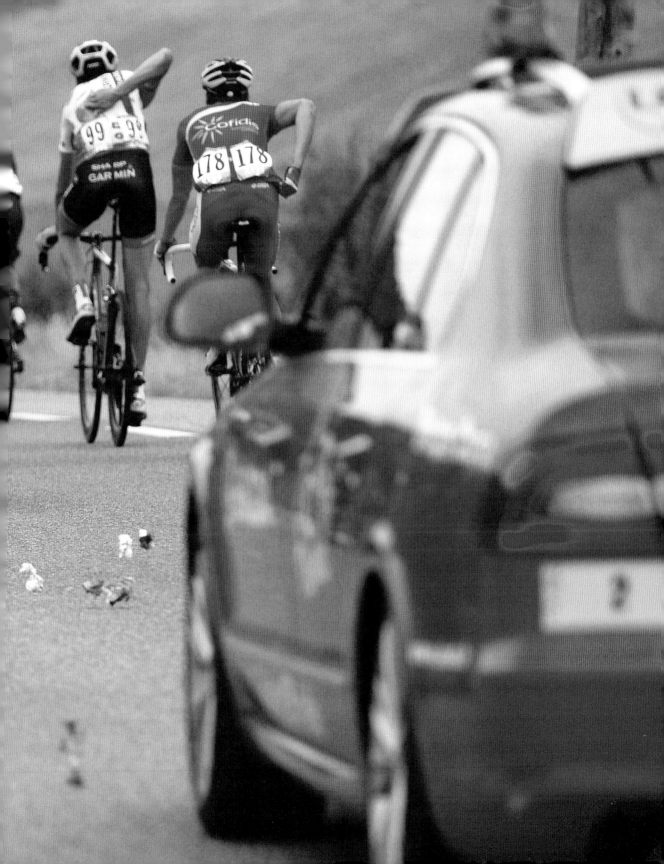

Short turbo session

For many amateur riders, myself included, a 60- to 90-minute blast on the turbo is a training staple during the week. Because of the relatively short duration of these sessions, many riders neglect to take on any fuel, which is a mistake. Although riding time is low, intensity is very high, and unless you take something on, your performance and resulting training gains will suffer. Eat well beforehand and don't forget that three- to four-hour window. During this type of workout you should be using gels or a carbohydrate sports drink. The latter is especially good as you'll be losing a lot of fluid on the turbo. Look to take on a gel, approximately halfway through the session and this should ensure that the second half isn't too hellish. Remember, you'll get a measurable boost just by having something sweet in your mouth. Because of the short duration of the session you don't need to worry about a recovery drink, but don't delay having your dinner too long.

Due to time constraints some riders will do their hard turbo session in the morning and struggle to fit in breakfast. I have found that actually having a recovery drink before a morning session (15–20 minutes before) helps to prepare the rider for the workout and feeds them during the session but is easily tolerated digestively. An ideal drink would be one that provides about 20 g of protein and about 30 g of carbohydrate.

Carbohydrate-fasted (metabolic) ride

Fasted training rides are very fashionable at the moment, but are nothing new. Roger Hammond used to do fasted rides as part of his early season training. The British former road cyclist would head out and, on his first go, bonk after maybe 90 minutes. Next time he might last for two hours before bonking and he'd just keep building up in this way. I personally do not like riders doing completely fasted rides, but I believe controlling carbohydrate intake in the right riding situations can be useful.

Science does seem to back up the rationale behind

carbohydrate-restricted training now. Your body will tend to use whatever fuel it has in abundance so, if you've got lots of carbohydrates in your blood and muscles, that's what your body will burn. By training with your body in a carbohydrate-fasted state, you force it to utilise fat as a fuel, making you a more efficient rider. What's important to remember is that this type of training is about increasing fat oxidation and efficiency, not weight loss. By improving your fat-burning ability, you'll conserve your carbohydrate reserves when you ride. This means you won't be so carbohydrate reliant and, if you struggle to take on board sufficient carbohydrate, you bonk. For pro riders, having excellent fat-burning ability is essential. A bike race is normally decided during the final 20–30 km and it's then, when the hammer goes down, that they really need some carbohydrate left in their system. Being able to tap into your fat reserves and save your carbohydrates for when you really need them will allow you to ride stronger for longer.

Current thinking is that there is no need to train in a completely fasted state, but instead that taking on some protein before heading out may actually enhance the training effect. Having an omelette or some yoghurt before riding will make the training less stressful on your immune system, your body will slowly convert some of the protein to blood sugar, making the ride more pleasant, and you'll recover faster from the session.

As with all rides, intensity is key and carbohydrate-fasted rides have to be ridden strictly in Zones 1 and 2. One of the problems with this type of training is that people can overdo the frequency, so every ride becomes a metabolic ride. This may help build endurance, but can massively effect the rider's ability to perform quality efforts. Remember, fuel for the ride and goals you want to achieve. Though it's a very time-effective way to increase your endurance and, because of the state it puts your body in, you can get the same benefits from a three-hour ride as you would from four hours, there's no need, however, to do the whole ride carbohydrate-fasted. Take something on, like a rice cake, which contains some protein too, and then fuel as you would on a regular steady-paced ride.

These rides can be built up: start by riding for 60–90 minutes before having any carbohydrates, then next time try two hours. If you are doing these for three hours or more, it's also worth having a bottle of protein to sip from the start of the ride. Look for a product, such as a quality whey protein, which will give you about 20 g of protein with minimal carbohydrate. Incidentally, if you commute to work by bike, making this a carbohydrate-fasted ride is a great way to get some training benefits.

HOW THE PROS FUEL THEIR RIDES

The table opposite shows a typical three-day training block for a professional rider. It illustrates how their nutrition is adapted to the demands and goals of the training session being performed. A three-day cycle of training is typical for professional riders. For most amateur riders it would be hard to find the time for this amount of training and longer rides are often tied to weekends, but some of the principles can be adapted. If you're going on a week's training camp, by following these principles and planning a bit, you'll get more out of it.

The first two days will include more intensity because the rider is still fresh from the rest day and muscle glycogen supplies are full. The third day may then be a metabolic day, designed to improve the body's ability to utilize body fat and conserve carbohydrate. Fuelling on the bike is therefore designed to support the training. On this plan, there is no recovery drink because the recovery meal is readily available, but if the recovery meal is delayed, the use of a recovery drink can be useful.

		Day 1	**Day 2**	**Day 3**
Aim of training		Increase capacity (aerobic power) and endurance	Build basic endurance and functional threshold	Build basic endurance and functional threshold Metabolic ride
Training		4 ½ hours: 60 min in zone 2, 3 x 5 min in zone 4 with 5 min easy between efforts, 15 min in zone 2, 3 x 5 min in zone 4 with 5 min easy between efforts, 90 min zone 2 (ride home)	5 hours: 90 min in zone 2; 3 x 20 min in zone 3 with 15 min recovery between each effort; 90 min in zone 2 (ride home)	5 hours: 30 min in zone 2–3, rest of ride in zone 1–2
Meal	Breakfast	Large bowl of porridge with seed and nut mix, 3 egg omelette, coffee	Large bowl of porridge with seed and nut mix; 3 egg omelette; coffee	3 egg omelette, ½ avocado, coffee
	On the bike	1 banana after 45 mins, 1 gel 5 mins before efforts, 1 caffeine gel after the first 3 efforts, 1 energy bar after the second 3 efforts, 2 bottles of energy drink, 2 bottles of water	1 banana after 45 mins, 1 gel 5 mins before each effort, 1 caffeine gel 5 mins before the last effort, 1 energy bar after last effort, 2 bottles of energy drink, 2 bottles of water	1 bottle of protein drink in first 60 mins, 1 banana after 90 mins, 4 bottles of water
		Total carbohydrate: approx. 180 g	Total carbohydrate: approx. 180 g	Total carbohydrate: 30 g Total protein: 20 g
	Recovery meal	Medium chicken breast, medium sweet potato, green salad with two tomatoes, olive oil and balsamic vinegar dressing	Tuna (one can), gnocchi, carrot and avocado salad with olive oil dressing	Chicken breast, 3–4 new potatoes, green salad including two tomatoes, olive oil and balsamic vinegar dressing
	Evening meal	Salmon steak (approx. 150 g), rice and quinoa (mixed), 200 g cooked mixed vegetables	Steak, sweet potato mash, carrots, broccoli	Pork steak, pasta and tomato sauce, spinach
	Evening snack	Natural yoghurt and honey	Natural yoghurt and honey	Natural yoghurt and honey

PRO STORY: BONKING ON ALPE D'HUEZ

In one of the defining moments of his 2013 Tour de France win, Chris Froome's blood-sugar crisis on Alpe d'Huez showed how bonking can happen to even the best riders and what to do if it happens to you. On the second ascent of the infamous Alpe that day, Chris put in a big effort to drop Alberto Contador and that pushed him over the edge. You could see it happening. He looked at his legs as if he was asking them what was going on, and he came to a near standstill. He would have still had some muscle glycogen left, but the high intensity he was riding at would have caused his blood sugar to suddenly drop and his brain would have initiated shut down. Fortunately, he had his loyal lieutenant, Richie Porte, riding with him and, despite incurring a 20-second penalty for taking food within the final 20 km, the two gels that he fetched for Chris from the team car saved the day. Richie gave Chris two pineapple juice-based gels that would have provided about 44 g of carbohydrate. There's no doubt in my mind that without those gels his losses would have been far more than 20 seconds. After that stage some people questioned this decision, saying at that point in the race the gels had no time to act and were a waste of time. However, just that sweetness in his mouth and on his tongue would have stimulated his brain and allowed more glucose to be released from his liver. If you watch a replay, you can see he took the gels and the effect was almost instantaneous. The lesson to learn from this is that, even if you're only 15 minutes from the end of a ride or race and starting to struggle, it's still worth taking a gel or having a good gulp of sports drink. If you bonk earlier on in a ride, take a gel or two, back right off the intensity and give your body a chance to recover. Once you're going again, don't make the same mistake: maybe ride a little easier and re-establish a disciplined regular fuelling routine.

KNOWLEDGE TO TAKE AWAY

- **Monitor intensity** *Riding intensity and nutrition are intrinsically linked so for optimal fuelling on the bike it is vital that you accurately monitor either heart rate or power.*

- **Tailor nutrition to the ride** *Adapt your nutrition to the demands of the ride and the training effects you want to attain. Adopt the same analytical and methodical approach to your nutrition as to the structure of your workouts.*

- **Be disciplined** *Never forget to fuel, set an alarm or put a note on your stem. Even pros have to do this so there's no shame in doing something similar.*

- **Try it in training** *Never try a new product for the first time at an event. Find out what the feed stations are providing and test it on some training rides.*

- **Beat the bonk** *It happens to the best riders, but even if you're near the end of a ride, just a bit of sweetness in your mouth will give you a genuine boost.*

RICE CAKES

··

These are now a staple for the whole pro peloton. They are super-easy to make and can provide a tasty snack for kids as well. I have used these in other endurance sports, including Olympic sailing.

Servings 20
Calories per serving:
    157 kcal
Carbohydrate per serving: 23 g
Fat per serving: 6 g
Protein per serving: 3 g

INGREDIENTS

500 g white short-grain rice
1 l water
2 tbsp coconut oil
2 tbsp sugar (white or brown)
1 tsp vanilla extract
300 g cream cheese (or
    200 g creamed coconut)

METHOD

1. In a rice cooker, cook the rice with the water, sugar, vanilla and coconut oil. If you are not using a rice cooker, follow the instructions on the rice packet.

2. When cooked, mix in the cream cheese. For a non-dairy alternative, substitute 200 g of creamed coconut.

3. Spoon into large zip-lock freezer bags and flatten and smooth the air out. Leave to cool on a flat tray and, once cool, refrigerate overnight.

4. Cut into small squares and store in an air-tight container in the fridge. They'll usually keep for about four days.

5. For on the bike, simply wrap the individual squares in foil.

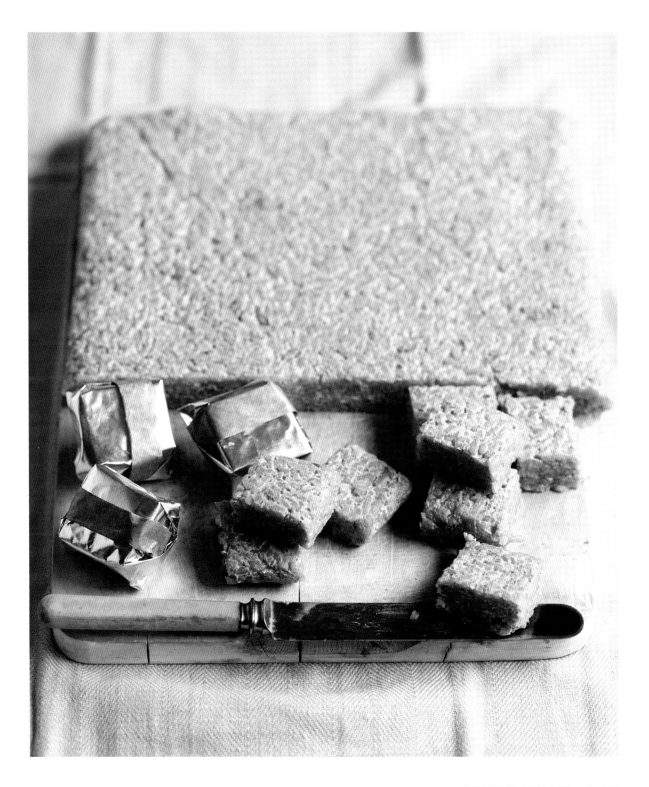

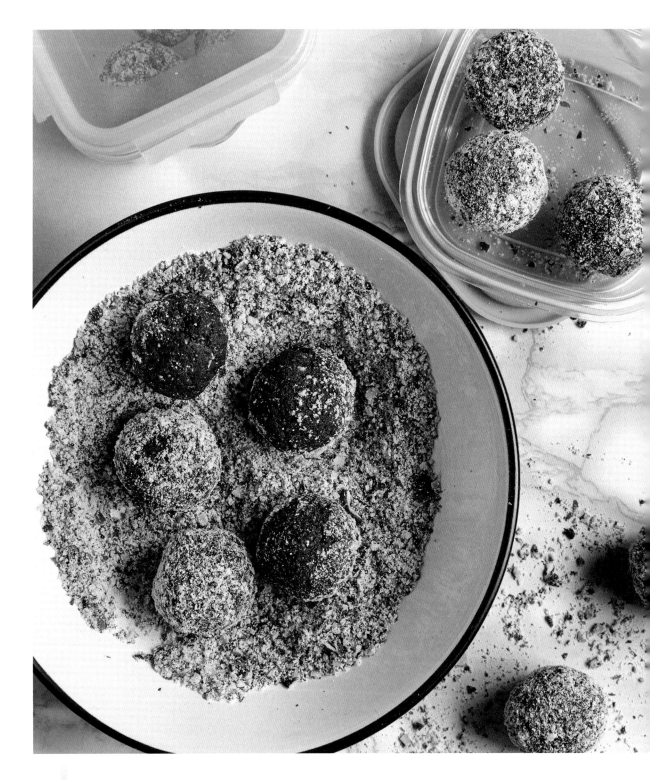

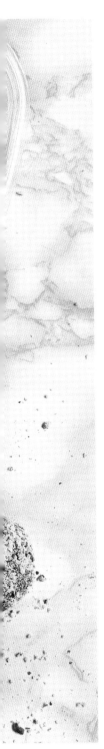

HOMEMADE ENERGY BALLS

··

These delicious energy balls are a great source of protein and, as well as being great on the bike, are brilliant for beating cravings between meals.

Servings 5
Calories per serving:
  195 kcal
Carbohydrate per serving: 26 g
Fat per serving: 9 g
Protein per serving: 7 g

INGREDIENTS

100 g dried dates
30 g rolled oat flakes
2 tbsp agave nectar syrup
24 g pumpkin seeds
1 tsp vanilla extract
1 tbsp cocoa powder
1 tbsp protein powder
  (optional)

METHOD

1. Place the pumpkin seeds into a blender and blitz until smooth, then spread out on a large plate.

2. Put the remaining ingredients in the blender and blend until you have a very smooth paste. With wet hands, remove the dough and form into walnut-sized balls.

3. Roll the balls in the blended pumpkin seeds. They will keep for about two weeks in an airtight container.

TRADITIONAL PANINI

'Panini' in Italian simply means 'sandwiches' and they are one of the most traditional cycling foods. They tend to be eaten in the earlier part of the race and are definitely in the 'lump of coal' end of the food spectrum. The traditional bread for these are doughy sweet Italian rolls, but I don't like these and tend to use a French baguette. The fillings can be really varied, but often combine both sweet and savoury, such as jam and cream cheese. Other popular fillings include ham, peanut butter and honey.

Serves 4
Calories per serving:
  163 kcal
Carbohydrate per serving: 22 g
Fat per serving: 3 g
Protein per serving: 3 g

INGREDIENTS
½ French baguette
100 g cream cheese
100 g jam

METHOD

1. Slice the baguette down the middle lengthways. Scoop out the soft dough to create a trough in the bread.

2. Spread the jam and cheese evenly in the trough.

3. Join the two sides of bread together and cut into 4–5 equal pieces.

4. Wrap and eat on the bike.

WRAP IT LIKE A PRO

One of the keys to eating well on the bike is making it as easy as possible. You don't want to waste time, or risk crashing, struggling to undo a wrapper. The soigneurs on pro teams realise this and are experts at wrapping on-the-bike snacks like rice cakes and paninis. Make sure you look for non-stick kitchen foil: Bacofoil is an easily available brand in the UK, as this folds the best, stays wrapped, but is easy to undo.

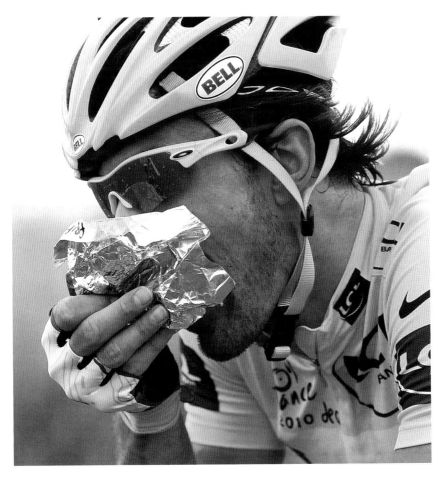

Fabian Cancellara with team Saxo Bank has a snack during stage six of the 2010 Tour de France

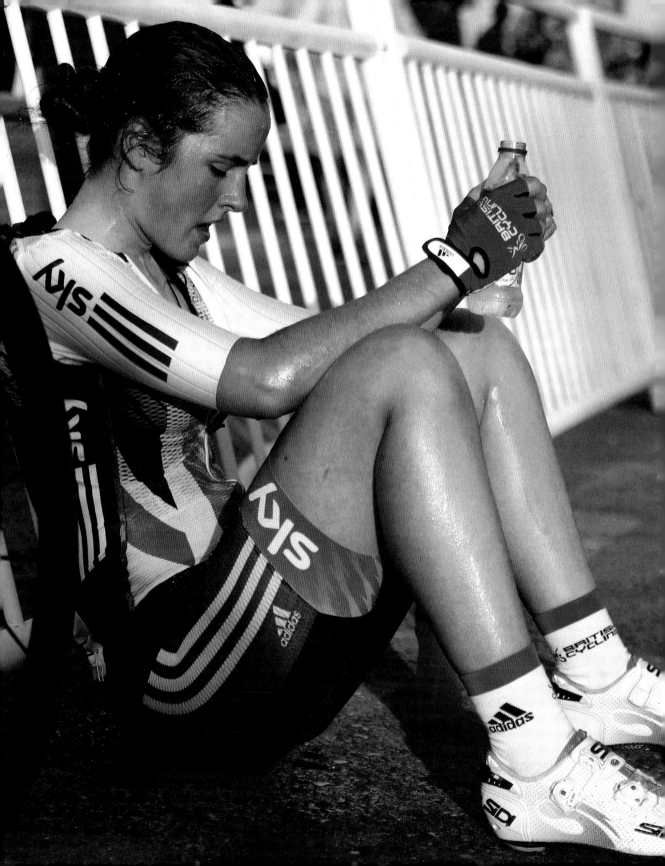

RECOVERY

We already started to touch on the subject of recovery in the last chapter, showing how, for certain rides, using a protein-rich recovery drink as you ride home and cool down can start the recovery process. However, as with fuelling during a ride, what and when you take on nutrition for recovery is dependent on the session you've just done, the training you've got planned in the next 24 hours and the availability of food. Optimising recovery post-training or post-racing is vitally important. It's said that Grand Tours aren't necessarily won by the strongest riders but by the ones who recover best. This doesn't mean though that you've got to have a carbohydrate and protein recovery drink after every single ride. For me, recovery is really about enabling the athlete to be able to perform again when they need to perform and how they need to perform.

TYPES OF RECOVERY

After a bike ride, there are three main types of recovery that your body undergoes and that you have to think about. These can be broadly thought of as metabolic, muscular (physiological) and psychological. Psychological recovery is the rider's emotional well-being and readiness to ride again. If it has been a particularly tough ride, it may take longer before you feel motivated to get out again. There is a big difference though between motivation and commitment. Motivation is saying 'I am going out to ride in the morning' or 'I am not going to eat more chocolate cake', but commitment is actually doing it. Sports psychology is a massively complex area of performance that is far beyond my personal area of expertise, but if you are struggling with this aspect of your riding, seeking the help of a qualified sports psychologist may be beneficial. This chapter, however, will focus on the metabolic and muscular aspects of recovery.

Annasley Park recovers after the Elite Women road race in the 2016 UCI Road World Championships

Metabolic recovery

Metabolic recovery is what we normally think of when we talk about recovery, but in actual fact it is not as important or necessary as you probably think. This is an energy recovery where you're replacing depleted carbohydrate stores in your body so that you have sufficient reserves in place for your next session. If you're not training or racing the next day, there isn't the urgency to take on board additional carbohydrates and you can easily overeat if you do. You'll often hear about a golden window of opportunity up to 20 minutes post exercise, where your body will hoover up any carbohydrates you provide and maximise your glycogen stores. The muscles have a limited capacity to store glycogen and the transport of carbohydrate into them is dependent on 'transporters' (Glute 4 transporters) being activated. These transporters are activated by insulin and/or vigorous exercise, which is why, post exercise, if the muscle is depleted, it can be most readily refilled. The problem with studies that showed this is that they used protocols which totally depleted the subjects' glycogen stores. For most rides and workouts, this simply shouldn't happen if you're training smart.

If you're fuelling well on the bike, the need to take on excessive carbohydrate immediately just isn't as crucial as many people think. One potential exception to this can be a long carbohydrate-fasted/metabolic ride (see Chapter 6), but for most amateur riders, only the first 90–120 minutes of such a ride would be completely carbohydrate-fasted and then they'd be fuelling normally. Another situation that amateur riders often encounter where carbohydrates are more important is if they're doing a double-session day. This will often be a turbo session or a hard ride into work in the morning and then maybe hitting the gym in the evening. After the morning workout some easily available carbohydrates would be advantageous. A final scenario would be if you misfuelled a ride, ended up bonking, heavily depleted your glycogen stores and were riding the next day. In all of these situations, you should be looking to consume 1 g of carbohydrate per kg of bodyweight as soon as you practically can after your ride. It's important to remember though that these are exceptions and that many commercially available recovery drinks deliver far more carbohydrates than you'll normally require.

Sometimes, when racing, the mountain domestiques of a GC contender will go full gas at the front of the line on a climb, to keep the pace high and to stop attacks. They will go as hard as they can until they literally can't go on and will then peel off. This is often referred to as 'emptying the tank' and is a situation where the rider will significantly deplete their glycogen reserves. It is a tactic that is often associated with Team Sky in mountain stages and that I had to take into consideration when refuelling the riders after a stage.

Even on Grand Tours, the recovery drink that the riders I work with will have immediately on finishing a stage tends to be predominately protein. This will supply about 20 g of whey protein, 5 g of glutamine and a couple of grams of leucine. They will have fuelled well on the bike and can eat the carbohydrates they require to top up their glycogen stores through the afternoon and evening. The riders prefer to eat the carbohydrates they need, usually in the form of rice. On mountain-top finishes, where the riders will have performed a 'tank-emptying' effort, we would add about 30 g of extra carbohydrate of plain maltodextrin, a long chain carbohydrate, to the protein drink.

Traditional thinking was that post-ride carbohydrates should have a high Glycemic Index so that they're quickly available to the body. There is some logic to this, but the problem is that high Glycemic Index carbohydrates also cause an insulin spike, which results in a high proportion of them being converted to and stored as fat. Unless you find yourself in one of the situations described above, where you are significantly glycogen depleted, you should look for lower Glycemic Index choices. As with all the nutritional decisions, what you choose should be determined by the training or racing you've just done and what you're planning to do next. If you have done a session that has depleted your glycogen and are training and racing again soon, taking on high Glycemic Index carbohydrates may be the best for you.

Muscular recovery

Muscular recovery is where protein, and more specifically the amino acids that are its building blocks, comes in. During the last 10 to 15 years we've really come to understand its importance to performance in endurance sports. As discussed in Chapter 1, all proteins are comprised arrangements of the 20 or so amino acids. Our bodies can synthesise most of these amino acids, but there are around eight, known as the essential amino acids, that have to be supplied by our diet. Animal source protein, such as meat, fish, eggs and dairy, will always contain all eight of these essential amino acids, which are said to be complete proteins. The majority of vegetable protein sources are incomplete, but by being aware of this and combining different sources, vegetarians and vegans can obtain their complete complement of amino acids.

When we exercise, we actually cause some of the proteins within our own bodies to start to break down and this is known as a catabolic response. Once we finish exercising, we're in a state where our bodies can rebuild and extend these proteins. This rebuilding process is referred to as an 'anabolic phase'. When you say anabolic, people automatically tend to think of anabolic steroids, bodybuilders and huge muscles, but, as an endurance athlete, this just isn't the case. When a bodybuilder trains, they'll stress their muscle fibres, which adapt by becoming bigger, but in endurance athletes the anabolic phase is subtler, though equally important. Within the cells of our muscles we have tiny powerhouses known as mitochondria, which are responsible for energy production. Endurance training stresses our muscles and stimulates them to create more mitochondria to cope with the additional load. This is all driven by the amino acids and protein that we supply. If we don't give our body the protein it requires

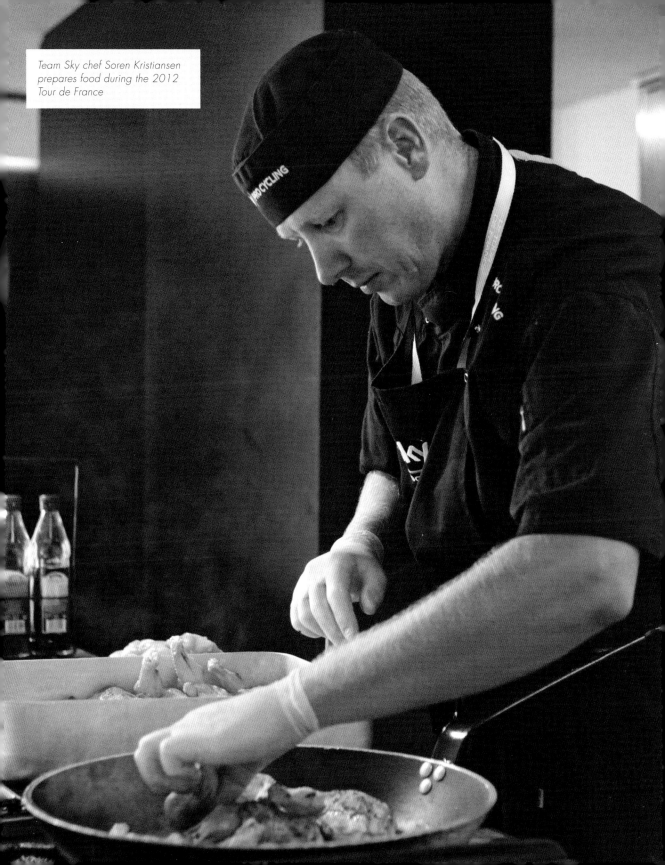

Team Sky chef Soren Kristiansen prepares food during the 2012 Tour de France

after exercise, it'll struggle to adapt. Through modern science we have a better understanding of the training effect and can see the muscle post exercise triggering certain genes that act like tiny messengers and inform the muscle to change.

Probably the easiest and quickest way to take some protein on post exercise is to consume protein powder shaken up into a drink. These powders are really nothing special though and are mainly dairy-based. During cheese production the milk is split into casein and whey. The casein forms the solid blocks and the whey, which is easily dissolved in water, is a straw-coloured solution. The composition of the amino acids in the whey and casein proteins is slightly different. The whey protein contains more of the branch chain amino acids, such as lucine, which have a greater effect on protein synthesis. In the past the whey would have been fed to pigs, but now it's freeze-dried and sold to athletes!

A protein drink is an incredibly effective way to kick-start your recovery after most rides, races and training sessions. That's why the first drink I'll give pro riders on a Grand Tour is predominately protein and then the riders will top up their carbohydrates with real food. A protein drink is also very good for rehydration, which is another key aspect of recovery. You should generally look to consume about 20 g of protein in 500 ml of water.

WHEN TO HAVE A RECOVERY DRINK

Many riders get confused about when they should be having a recovery drink. It's not uncommon for riders to double up, necking a recovery drink and then tucking into lunch or dinner immediately afterwards. This won't help you to recover any quicker and certainly won't do your waistline any good. The times when you should be using a recovery drink are when you've done some hard training or a race and are not going to be able to have a meal for 60–90 minutes. An example might be heading out for a long training ride at 10 a.m., not getting back until 3 p.m., effectively missing lunch while you're riding and then not having your main meal until 6 p.m. This is when a recovery drink is really useful to have either during the cool-down phase of the ride or as soon as you get home. It will then kick-start and support your recovery up until you have your evening meal. Remember, if you've fuelled properly on the bike, you won't have depleted your glycogen stores so protein is your priority and you can eat the carbohydrates that you do require with your meal. Another suitable time could be after a race when you're travelling home and it will take a couple of hours before you're able to have a decent meal. Sessions such as an evening track league can create a challenge as you may not finish racing until 9 p.m. and then not get home until 10 p.m., so a recovery drink after the track league followed by a bowl of cereal when you get home is a good option.

FOODS TO BOOST RECOVERY

A certain amount of inflammation or stress is part of the training and adaptation process which leads to us becoming fitter and stronger. Training puts your body under duress so it either adapts and improves or breaks down. The idea is to put enough load on the body not to cause breakdown, but to still provide the stimulation for adaptation. Good nutrition plays a key role in keeping a rider on the right side of this balance and for fuelling the adaptations. Foods with antioxidant and anti-inflammatory properties can help us recover from tough workouts or races; look for brightly coloured foods – tomatoes and peppers are brilliant. If you just use recovery drinks, rather than eating real foods, you'll be missing out on some of these natural recovery agents, such as polyphenols. This is one of the reasons I use a lot of vegetable and fruit juices with riders as it's an easy way to get these nutrients without having to consume large volumes of whole fruits and vegetables, which can be stressful on the gut.

It's also important to remember that fats play an important role in recovery but many endurance athletes are 'fat phobic'. Some fats, however, such as the omega-3 fats found in fish oils, can really help to regulate some of the excessive stress and inflammation that we get from very hard exercise. Fats play a vital role in our inflammatory and stress system. It's not that the omega-3 fats are actually anti-inflammatories, like ibuprofen, it's more that they give the body a helping hand in dealing with and recovering from the inflammation. If there is too much physiological stress, the recovery from training and racing is impeded. Modern diets tend to be low in omega-3 fats, so this is why supplements can be useful. The actual fat that we believe is key is eicosapentaenoic acid (EPA).

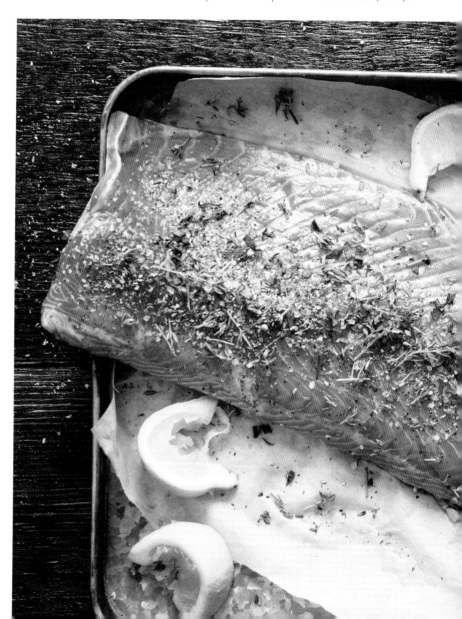

It's not actually the fish that make these fats, it's the krill that the fish feed on. These fats not only reduce some of the stress from training, they may also even increase the protein synthesis that's crucial to recovery and adaptation. Increasing omega-3 intake is something that I recommend to all pro riders and serious amateurs and you should aim to consume 2 g per day of a high-quality EPA oil. If you struggle with the taste of the pure oil, you can always choose capsules.

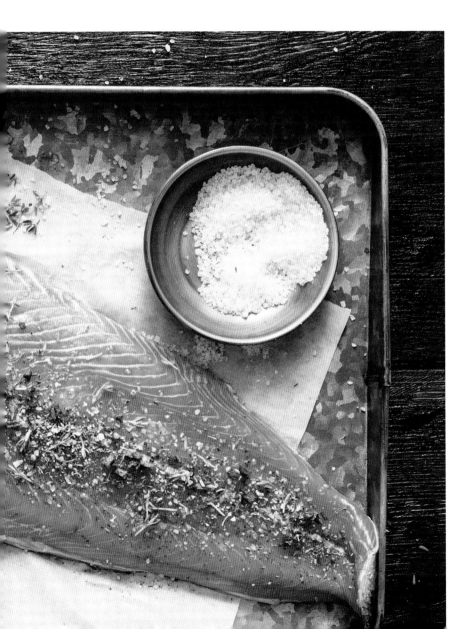

EATING ON REST DAYS

All riders struggle with managing their nutrition on rest days, pros especially as they get bored, but it's really about re-establishing the body's balance, providing it with the nutrients for both metabolic and muscular recovery and preparing it for the next block of training. You don't need to overeat to achieve this, you simply need to stick to your normal meal plan of breakfast, lunch and dinner, maybe with mid-morning and mid-afternoon snacks of a piece of fruit or some nuts. You can probably slightly reduce your carbohydrate portions. As you'll not have ridden and had lunch off the bike, your evening meal should be smaller as the total amount you eat will naturally need to be dialled down.

Below is a typical rest day diet for a pro rider which follows on from the three-day training block we looked at in the previous chapter. Although it's called a rest day, the riders will still usually go out for a very easy-paced 60- to 90-minute ride.

Meal	Food
Breakfast	Small bowl of porridge, natural yoghurt with blueberries, coffee
Snack on the bike	Banana
Lunch	Salmon steak, medium sweet potato and mixed green salad
Snack	Coffee and a piece of cake
Evening meal	Steak, risotto, broccoli, carrots. Yoghurt and honey
Evening snack	Hot chocolate

PRO STORY: RECOVERING FOR GOLD

In a three-week long Grand Tour, where one bad day can see a rider tumble down the GC, recovery is crucial. In 2012, when Sir Bradley Wiggins won the Tour de France, as other riders faded, he grew stronger and dominated the final time trial. An even more amazing feat of recovery followed when, a week later, he went on to take gold in the Olympic time trial. This was not only testament to his incredible ability, discipline and focus as an athlete, but to the many measures that both Team Sky and British Cycling put in place to optimise his recovery. One of these, which at the time still wasn't 100 per cent accepted in cycling, was the importance of consuming protein after riding. However, as other teams witnessed our riders seemingly getting stronger as theirs started to fade, it wasn't long before a greater emphasis on the importance of protein became the norm.

Another example of changing the way things had always been done was getting rid of post-stage sodas. When I started in pro cycling it was the norm for riders to have a can of soda, such as cola, at the end of the stage. You'd give them a bag with a can of cola and a recovery drink in it, and most of the time the recovery drink would be left untouched. Apart from giving the body some sugar and water, cola does little for recovery. In fact, it may undermine the recovery process because the soda is so acidic and may affect gut health. One of the first things we did at Team Sky was to stop giving the riders the soda. They weren't happy at first, but once we explained the reasons behind it, they accepted it.

HOW TO MAXIMISE YOUR RECOVERY

Along with getting your nutrition right, there are a number of other steps you can take, and some to avoid, to maximise your recovery from tough rides.

Sleep

If you're not sleeping well or not getting enough sleep, your recovery and adaptation to training will suffer. Long-term poor sleep will also result in diminished mental performance and an increase in the body's stress hormone cortisol. At Team Sky we realised the importance of our riders sleeping well on Grand Tours and went to the extreme of taking our own bedding and pillows to use in the hotels we stayed at.

Try to get into a bedtime routine that is conducive to sleep. Avoid caffeine after 3 p.m., alcohol and excessive screen time before going to bed. Don't perform hard workouts within a couple of hours of going to bed and make sure that your bedroom is well aired, at a comfortable temperature and properly dark. Finally, don't forget the calming camomile tea with honey that I recommend before heading to bed.

Stretching

The benefit of stretching is still a fairly controversial and debated area in sports science. However, once you are showered and relaxed, some gentle stretching or yoga or can definitely help to ease out some of the tightness felt after a hard ride or even after a long day sat at a desk.

Elevate

It'd be great if we could all live our lives by the pro cyclist mantra of 'Never stand when you can sit and never sit when you can lie down'. It's funny how, when I am with cyclists who may have ridden 200 km that day, they would never dream of walking up a flight of stairs and would always get the lift. Unfortunately, work and family life make such a privileged existence impossible for non-pros. But if you can, after a hard ride, spend some time with your legs elevated as this can help recovery by promoting blood flow and aiding venous return to the heart. Lying with your head on a pillow and your legs up against a wall for five to ten minutes feels blissful and also gives you a gentle hamstring and lower-back stretch.

Massage

Despite not having irrefutable scientific support, if you ever tried to put an end to post-race rub-downs, you'd have a mass rider walkout. The overwhelming anecdotal evidence is that riders believe them to be an essential part of their recovery routine. A daily or even weekly massage is probably beyond the budgets of most amateur riders, but how about booking one in during recovery weeks or after a big event? Look for a qualified sports massage therapist with experience of treating cyclists and view it like a regular MOT for your body. They'll be able to identify any problematic areas and give you exercises or stretches to do to manage them. A good DIY massage option is to use a foam roller; you can even get small travel versions that fit easily into a suitcase.

Compression

Although the scientific evidence for performance gain and injury prevention is inconclusive, for recovery, compression clothing does seem to help. Putting on a pair of compression tights while you relax after a hard ride is certainly no hardship and I swear by them when travelling. Look for a medical-grade product with graduated compression and make sure the fit is spot-on.

Riding

On a rest day on a Grand Tour the riders will usually head out for a few hours of very easy-paced riding. Along with stopping them from getting bored, it helps prevent their legs from stiffening up and means that the next day's racing isn't too much of a shock. Some

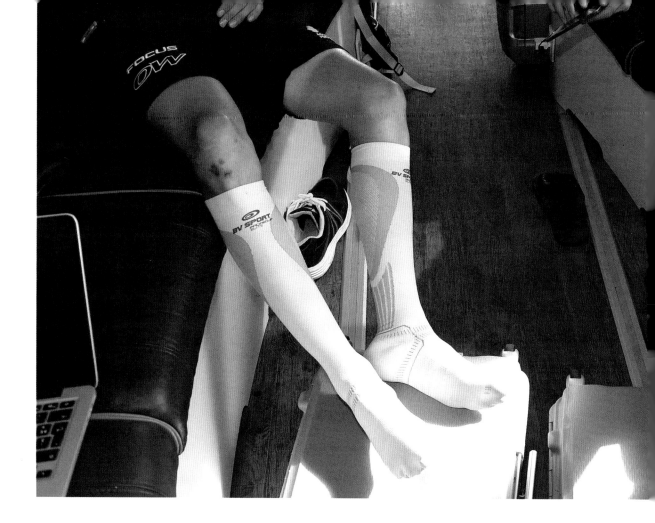

light riding definitely aids recovery, but it has to be genuinely light. Keep your bike in the small chainring, stay on the flat and stick to strict Zone 1. You should be applying minimal force through your pedal; imagine your cranks are made of glass. If you think you'll struggle to do this out on the road, rollers are a great option for a recovery spin.

Skip the ice bath

The good news is that ice baths have been shown to have very little benefit to recovery. For contact sports, such as rugby, they're useful for dealing with acute inflammation from impact, but for endurance activities such as cycling, reducing the inflammation

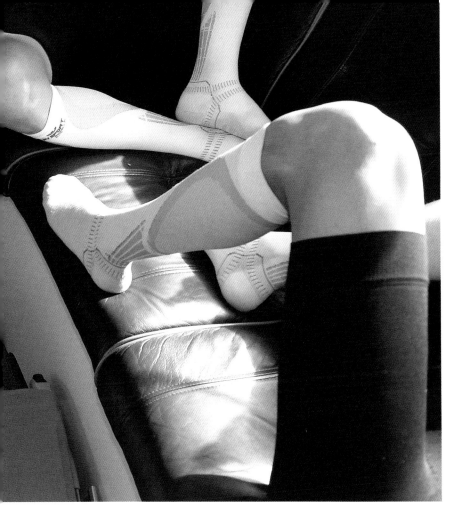

Team AG2R La Mondiale of France wearing decompression recovery socks during the 2016 Vuelta a España

in the muscles can actually lower the training stimulus. Enjoy your post-ride hot bath or shower guilt-free!

Avoid painkillers/anti-inflammatories

Although fairly commonplace, using non-steroidal anti-inflammatories, such as ibuprofen, during or after endurance activities isn't a good idea. Like ice baths, it'll reduce the positive inflammation response to training that stimulates your muscles to adapt and become stronger. More importantly though, they can have a negative effect on your stomach, potentially affecting digestion and kidney function.

KNOWLEDGE TO TAKE AWAY

- **Your riding dictates your fuelling** As with what you eat before and during your rides, what you consume post-ride should be determined by the ride you've just done, the exercise demands of the next 24 hours and the availability of food to you.

- **Metabolic recovery** This type of recovery replenishes your body's carbohydrate reserves, but in most circumstances if you've been fuelling well on the bike, these shouldn't be significantly depleted so there's no need to replenish urgently or excessively.

- **Muscular recovery** This type of recovery gives your muscles the fuel they need – protein – to adapt to the training they're doing. For strength and power athletes, this will be growth; for endurance athletes, it's an increase in mitochondria, the powerhouses of cells.

- **Don't stress about the '20-minute window of opportunity'** The studies showing this effect were performed on pre-fasted and totally glycogen-depleted subjects. You'll rarely, if ever, be in this state during your cycling training and racing.

- **Protein is king** Prioritise protein post-ride. If you're not going to be able to eat properly for more than 60–90 minutes after you finish, this is the time to reach for a protein shake. Look to have 20 g of protein in 500 ml of water. You can eat your carbohydrates as real food as part of your meal.

- **Don't forget quality fats** Don't fear fats. Omega-3 fats, especially eicosapentanoic acid (EPA), will help support your recovery. Remember, other good sources of fats include nuts, seeds and avocados.

DIY RECOVERY DRINK

There are lots of variations you can blend up, including adding fresh fruit, but this one is a convenient powder which can be easily made up after a race or training. You can add more carbohydrates by including maltodextrin (available from most pharmacists and sports nutrition companies). The nutritional information below does not include the extra carbohydrates, but if you add 20 g it will give about 20 g more of carbohydrates and 80 kcal.

Serves 1
Calories per serving:
   257 kcal
Carbohydrate per serving: 42 g
Fat per serving: 0.5 g
Protein per serving: 20 g

INGREDIENTS

60 g plain skimmed milk
   powder
500 ml water
2 tbsp milkshake flavouring

METHOD

1. It doesn't get simpler: just put the milk powder, milkshake flavouring and water in a shaker and give it a good shake.

2. If you make it up beforehand, keep it in a cold box or fridge

SLOW COOKER RECOVERY STEW

I find the slow cooker an invaluable piece of kitchen kit. Most houses have one but it probably sits in the cupboard unused. It's brilliant because you can just throw in all of the ingredients, go out for a ride or to work and then come home to a great-smelling house and a delicious meal.

Serves 6
Calories per serving:
   350 kcal
Carbohydrate per serving: 20 g
Fat per serving: 7.3 g
Protein per serving: 39 g

INGREDIENTS

1 kg thin beef or stewing
   steak, diced
200 g carrots, chopped
50 g canned lentils
200 g potatoes, peeled
   and diced
100 g onions, finely chopped
100 g canned split peas
400 g can chopped tomatoes
1 tbsp mixed herbs
2 bay leaves
250 ml water, extra if needed
Salt and pepper, to taste

METHOD

1. This is as easy as cooking gets. Throw all the ingredients into the slow cooker. Give them a stir and switch on to a medium heat and cook for 4–8 hours.

2. You may need to add a little more fluid and give the occasional stir but it's not usually necessary.

There's plenty here for several meals and you can always freeze some portions. Instead of the beef you can use chicken thighs; thighs hold together better than breast, but remember to remove the skin before cooking.

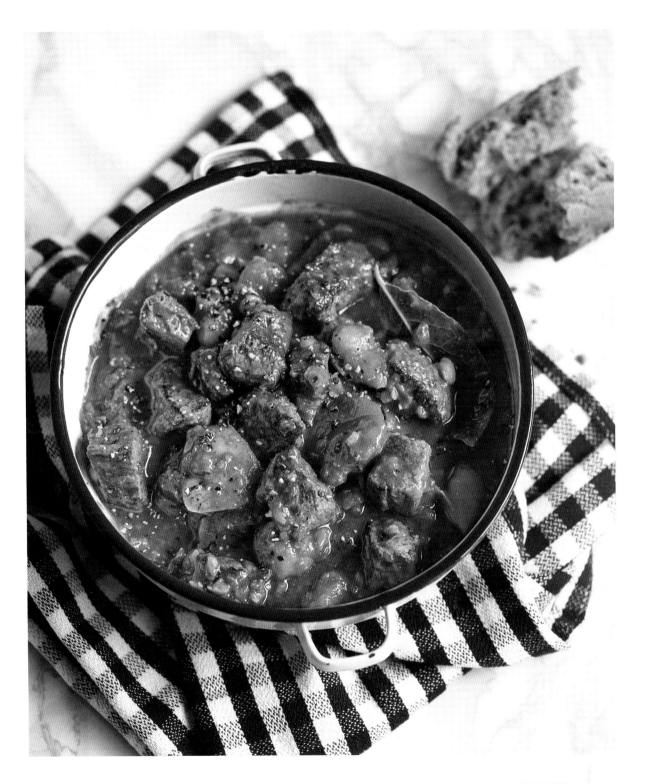

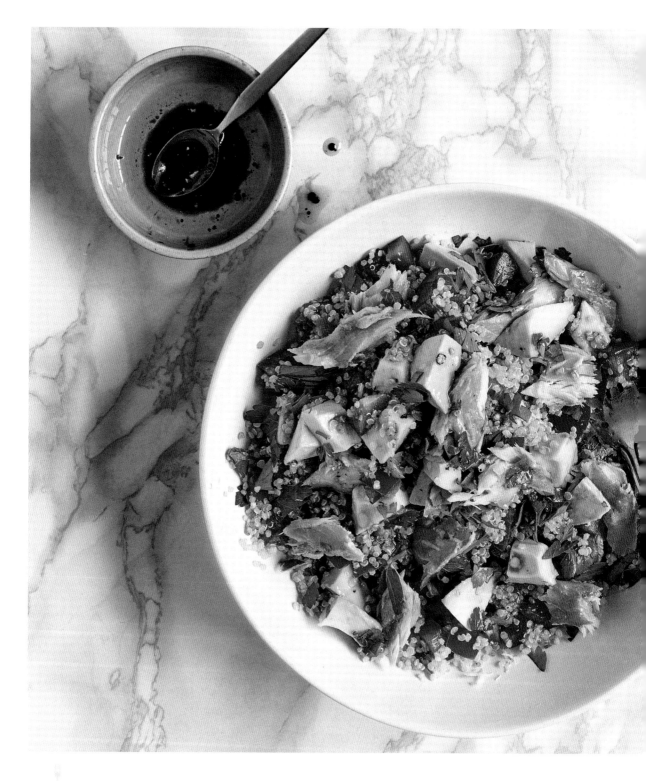

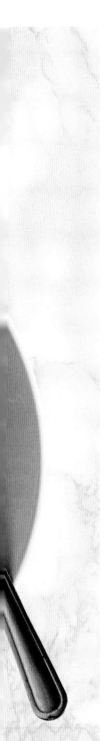

RECOVERY-BOOSTING MACKEREL AND TOMATO SALAD

Salads are a brilliant option for post-ride. They're quick to make and are great during the summer when you may not fancy a hot and heavy meal. This simple recipe is packed with healthy omega-3 fats from the mackerel and avocado, and moderate in carbs and high in protein.

Serves 1
Calories per serving:
   602 kcal
Carbohydrate per serving: 26 g
Fat per serving: 55 g
Protein per serving: 29 g

INGREDIENTS

1 smoked mackerel fillet
½ avocado
100 g quinoa, cooked
2 medium tomatoes
½ red pepper
Salt and pepper, to taste
Olive oil and Balsamic
   vinegar, if liked
Sprig of parsley, chopped

METHOD

1. Pre-cook the quinoa according to the packet instructions and allow to cool, or, for the ultimate easy meal, use a pre-cooked sachet.

2. Chop all the other ingredients. Remove the stone from the avocado and chop into small pieces.

3. Place in a large bowl, season and toss. Add some olive oil and Balsamic vinegar to dress if liked, and a scattering of chopped parsley to finish.

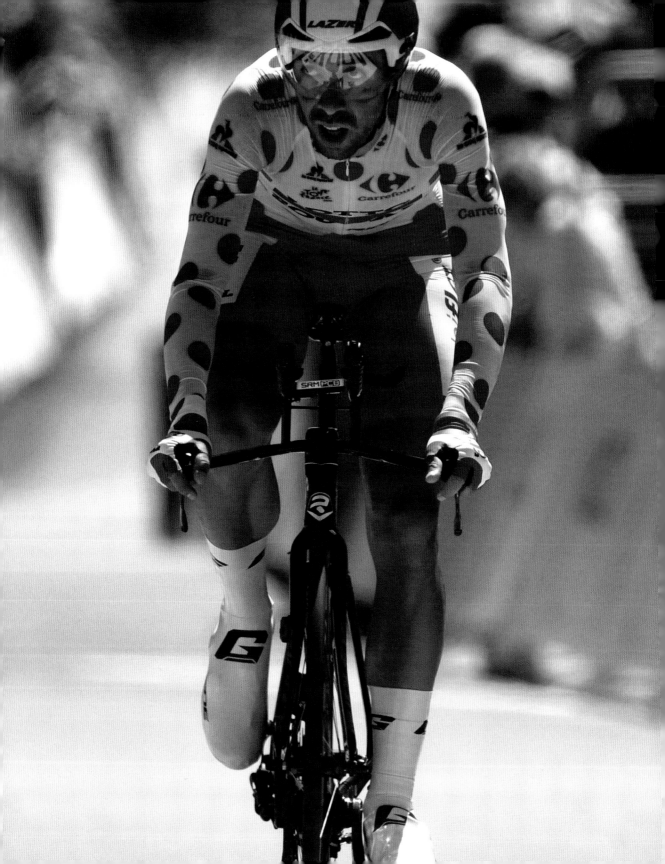

WEIGHT MANAGEMENT

If you watch the Tour de France, or any top-level bike race with significant climbs, you can guarantee that the podium contenders will all be whippet thin. Also, cycling magazines regularly churn out weight-loss tips, diets and advice so it's easy to think that you have to be super-skinny to be a successful cyclist. Although trimming a few pounds off your waistline will certainly be cheaper than trying to shave the same amount of weight off your bike with expensive component upgrades, first you need to think about your cycling goals. If you're a time trialist who mainly races on flat drag-strip courses, a track rider or even a circuit/crit rider, as long as you're not overweight, you're not really going to get much of a return on the effort you'd have to put in to shift a kilogram or two. In fact, if you lose too much, you'll start seeing your power drop and performance decrease. However, if you're targeting hilly races or sportives, or if you're a multisport athlete who has to run too, then weight does become more critical. On a 6 per cent incline it's estimated that a rider will typically save 5 watts (this is about 4 seconds per km) for every kilogram of weight, so it's easy to see why, if you're riding hills, you don't want to be carrying any extra ballast. Weight loss isn't a shortcut to performance though and you definitely shouldn't be trying to crash weight off to make up for a lack of training and preparation.

BODY COMPOSITION

One of the first things I do when starting work with an athlete is to try and establish an idea of their body composition. From this we can find out their lean mass, in particular muscle mass, but also bones and organs, and their fat mass.

In simple terms we can think of two classes of body fat. The first is storage fat, which the body has in place as an energy source. This can be further crudely divided into the muscle triglyceride, fat stored in the muscles, and the more obvious

Thomas De Gendt, wearing the best climber's polka dot jersey, crosses the finish line of the 13th stage of the 2016 Tour de France

subcutaneous fat store under the skin. All of this fat is there and available to us as stored energy. The fat in the muscle provides working energy and, during long bouts of exercise or when you are fasting, the body mobilises the fats from the subcutaneous stores to act as a fuel source. Our body's tendency to store fat and stubbornly cling to it hails back to our evolutionary past. If you don't know when you'll make your next mammoth kill, having a backup energy store makes a lot of sense. This evolved survival mechanism of storing fat remains and, sadly, our bodies aren't aware that we want to lose fat to fit into a swimming costume or climb well on a bike, or that we have food in abundance. Even a lean person will have up to 10 kg (22 lb) of stored fat, which would provide the body with about 90,000 kcal. If you've ever wondered why we store excess energy as fat, the reason is pretty simple: fat is the most energy-dense nutrient. One gram of fat provides about 9 kcal/g of energy, whereas both protein and carbohydrate only provide about 4 kcal/g. Therefore, fat is the most efficient energy store. The second type of body fat is essential fat, which is found throughout the body. Every cell has fat in it. Fat provides protection for our organs, pads our feet and is necessary for the synthesis of many hormones.

Most athletes will want to lose fat mass, although there are cases where they'll drop lean mass too. An example of this was when Sir Bradley Wiggins switched from the track to road cycling and had to drop 8–9 kg (17.6–19.8 lb), some of which was lean mass. He's now gone back the other way, bulked up again to give him the power necessary for the team pursuit on the track and this has obviously worked, with the team taking gold and setting a World Record in Rio in 2016. However, for any body weight changes, unless you know your body composition, you're really working blind. There are a lot of methods of estimating body composition, including body pods which you sit in, scales that pass an electrical current through your body, known as bio-impedance, and skin-fold callipers. Techniques such as DEXA (dual-energy

X-ray absorptiometry) scans, an advanced version of an X-ray, are becoming more popular but they still rely on regression equations to produce their results. These equations use data from previous studies and, by applying it to the scan results, produce an estimate of body composition. It's important to remember this and, no matter how high-tech the kit looks, it's still reliant on these equations and is therefore only an estimate. I find these scans more useful for tracking changes in lean tissue and bone density rather than for deducing body-fat percentages. Similarly, the percentage body-fat figure that bio-impedance scales give tends to be wildly inaccurate as it's massively affected by factors such as hydration level.

My personal choice for tracking a rider's body composition is to measure skin folds at eight sites around the body. There are equations and tables that allow you to convert the skin folds total to a percentage figure, but I prefer to stick to and work from a sum of the skin folds. The percentage figure, again calculated using regression equations, will always only be an estimate and can easily give a false idea to an athlete about the amount of fat they can or can't lose. One formula or table might give an athlete 10 per cent body fat but, using a different one, they'll come out at 15 per cent.

By just using the sum of the sites and measuring at regular intervals of four to eight weeks, I can track an athlete's progress and form a good idea of the fat mass that they'll be able to lose. For a Grand Tour GC contender, I'd be looking for a total over the eight skin-fold sites of below 34–35 mm. For a Grand Tour domestique, who'll be having to do more work on the flat, it would be about 40 mm. To put that in perspective, a professional footballer would probably be in the region of 55–75 mm. Female athletes tend to be about 20 mm higher than their male counterparts. Women typically have more fat as an evolved adaption to child rearing as it provides a source of fuel for a growing foetus or dependent youngster if food supplies run low.

Most qualified personal trainers at your local gym should be

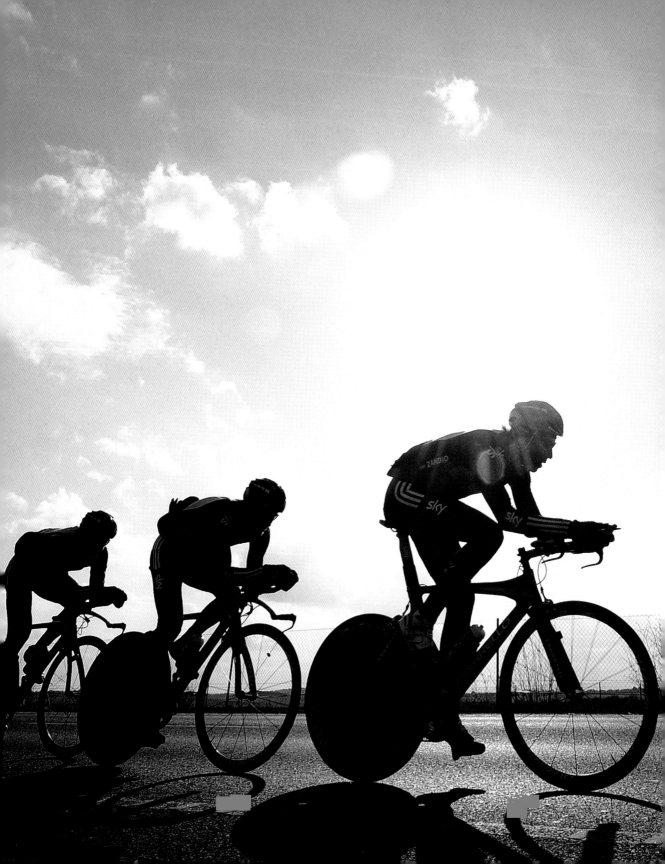

able to perform an eight-site skin-fold assessment. However, it's vital that the measurements are consistent and performed by the same individual each time. Remember though that it's the skin folds total you're interested in, not the percentage figure from them.

Scales do lie

What most people have at home is a set of bathroom scales. These can be useful for tracking weight, but they don't give you any information about what the weight you're gaining or losing consists of. Many people will put themselves on a diet and training regime, see the scales dropping and think they're doing a great job of losing fat. However, if your diet is too extreme and you're not providing your body with enough fuel, you'll be losing muscle mass along with fat. This comes back to our evolutionary past we previously discussed. As far as our body is concerned, a restrictive diet is a famine and it will do its utmost to maintain our fat reserves. Because we need to maintain brain function, and our brains are glucose dependent, however, our bodies can't convert body fat into glucose for the brain, but they can break down protein to provide it. The body's easily available protein source is its muscles and so it starts to destroy them. Another downside of this is that, by losing muscle mass, our metabolic rate drops, meaning our overall calorific need, even when at rest, is less. This explains why many people end up in an endless cycle of yo-yo dieting and always seem to put back on the weight they lost plus a little bit more.

Another survival mechanism that our evolutionary past has given us is that, in a starved state, our body can produce chemicals known as ketones from the breakdown of fat. The brain is able to use ketones as a fuel, but they take a good few hours to produce and give you unpleasant pear drop sweet-smelling breath. The Atkins Diet is a ketogenic diet which is designed, by eliminating carbohydrates entirely, to put the body in a catabolic (breaking down tissue) state. However, much of the weight loss seen will be muscle and water weight, along with fat. There have been reports in the media over the last few years about the use of ketones as a sports supplement, the theory being that if you ingested ketones, they could be used as an additional fuel source. Effective ketone supplements are some way off being commercially available due to issues with cost, taste, gastric tolerance and the massive salt load needed to get an effective dose. However, rumours are rife that some professional teams are already using them.

In 2004, I did some work with amateur boxers and the accepted wisdom then was, in the run-up to a competition, to really up their training and severely restrict food to make their weight. What I observed when monitoring their skin-fold measurements and weight was that, although their weight would drop by 3–4 kg (6.6–8.8 lb), the skin-folds sum wouldn't change. This meant that almost all of the weight they were losing was comprised of fluid and lean tissue. In an amateur boxing competition, which takes place over a number of days, this type of weight loss meant that they'd simply be getting weaker and weaker. By adopting a longer-term view to making their fighting weight, upping protein intake to preserve lean mass and not having to crash diet to lose weight at the last minute, they were able to minimise this performance drop-off.

Do weigh yourself to track your weight, but only in combination with skin-fold measurements. That way you'll know what any changes in weight really signify. Weigh yourself twice each week, trying to stick to the same time of day and either naked or wearing the same clothes each time.

You can also make use of scales to track hydration levels. If you weigh yourself daily and notice a sudden weight loss, especially if you've done a hard ride the day before, it's likely that you're dehydrated.

ENERGY BALANCE

Energy balance is a crude estimate of total energy of food coming into our bodies versus the energy we expend. If our energy balance is positive (i.e. we're consuming more than we're using), we'll gain weight, and conversely if we're expending more than we're consuming, we'll lose weight. With pro riders on a Grand Tour, I'll be aiming for them to maintain a neutral energy balance. They'll be coming into the race very lean and if they start losing more weight, it'll weaken them, but I also don't want them gaining fat as the race goes on.

When people are trying to work out what their daily calorific need is they often get confused. The first figure that contributes to it is your Basal Metabolic Rate (BMR) and this is simply the energy your body needs to exist. On top of this is the energy required for you to go about your day-to-day life, working, looking after the kids or doing some DIY, for example. Finally, as an athlete, there is the energy required to fuel your training. There are numerous calculators and online apps that supposedly allow you to work out your total energy requirement, but at best they're a rough estimate. Even when it comes to totalling up the energy you've expended in training, they often forget one crucial factor: as you become fitter, you become more efficient and use less energy, and very few models take this into account. Be wary of estimates of the calorie burn from exercise, even if you use a heart rate monitor as they tend to be significantly out. As discussed in Chapter 6, power meters provide much more reliable data concerning energy expenditure and, as their software becomes more sophisticated, this is only going to improve.

I've found that, although you can get a ballpark theoretical figure, a more functional approach to energy requirements is far better. I'll monitor body composition, weight, training load and diet and see how they affect one another in any individual rider. Once a data trend starts appearing, I can then tweak the rider's intake to achieve the goals we want. This may take a bit more time but in the long term it is far more effective than attempting to diet to arbitrary calorie targets.

You can do the same for yourself without a live-in nutritionist.

Use one of the online calculators to obtain a rough estimate of your caloric need, log your calorie intake and record the estimated calorie burn from your training. Having measured your skin folds and weighed yourself, follow these estimates and try to hit a negative energy balance of 500 kcal per day for about four weeks. See how your weight changes by weighing yourself twice a week and plotting the results. After four weeks, have your skin folds remeasured. If neither skin fold measurements nor weight are dropping, reduce your calorie intake slightly and/ or up your training. If your weight is dropping but your skin-fold measurements are staying the same, you're losing lean mass and need to increase your calorie consumption. If your weight is staying the same or dropping by about 0.5 kg (1.1 lb) per week, but skin-folds are falling, you're losing fat and retaining lean mass, which is ideal. Make the necessary tweaks to your energy balance depending on what you observe and keep reassessing.

One kilogram of body fat is worth about 7000 kcal, so, to lose a kilogram, you need to achieve this energy deficit. From a cycling point of view, if you're out riding at Zone 2 endurance intensity, you'll burn approximately 600 kcal/ hr and would therefore require just under 12 hours. This obviously doesn't take into account the fuel you consume while riding, so to lose fat from exercise alone takes an awful lot of work. You clearly have to make some modifications to your diet to try and achieve a consistent negative energy balance of about 500 kcal per day. It's not a lot to work with and an easy target to miss, especially with training to factor in. On a long ride day you might be well over this 500 kcal deficit and struggle to eat enough calories to bring you up to it, but it's important you do or you risk sacrificing lean tissue. Conversely, if you're having a rest day, the food you're allowed can seem meagre. Again, this is why a personalised approach – monitoring body composition and making appropriate tweaks to diet and training – is far better than following arbitrary calorie targets.

ADVICE FOR LOSING WEIGHT CORRECTLY

Heavy training isn't the time to lose weight

One mistake a lot of riders make is to try and lose weight during a heavy training block. This is really hard as your body needs the energy to train and without it, you'll be compromising the training you're doing. You've got to plan your fuelling based on the training you're doing and if you're putting in hard efforts, you need adequate fuel. Think strategically about your nutrition and training. If you've got a key event three to six months away and you feel that you could benefit by losing some body fat, look at achieving that fat loss early on when you'll probably be focusing on lower-intensity endurance work. If you leave it until late in your training, when you'll be wanting to add some higher-end fitness and work at a greater intensity, you'll really struggle. Occasionally a pro rider may have to drop a few kilos in the lead-up to a race, but it takes an awful lot of discipline and planning. We'll fuel precisely to the workouts they're doing, just providing enough energy to complete their efforts. It's a lot easier for them and me if they come back from the off-season close to their racing weight! In this situation, the carbohydrate component of the diet is mainly given around training, at breakfast, as a gel for efforts on the bike and then the recovery meal. The evening meal will be lighter in carbs and about half the size of the lunchtime recovery meal. When I have a rider really pushing to lose weight, I never compromise protein or fats. Fats are so important for the hormonal and numerous other vital functions of the body.

There are potentially real health risks of chronic low-energy intake, particularly to bone health. Bones are fascinating organs in the body. Most people see them as just structural to keep the body from flopping around like a blob of jelly, but in fact bones

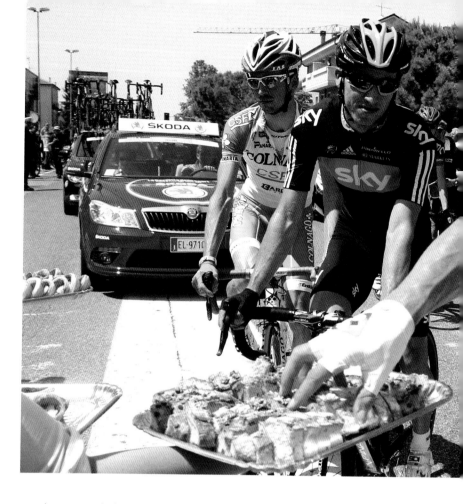

are living and dynamic tissue in a constant flux of re-modelling. It can be thought of as a protein lattice filled with minerals such as calcium and phosphate. Athletes with low-energy intakes can risk compromising the density of their bones. The bone health paradox is complicated because bone health is affected by so many factors; one of which is vitamin D status (see page 20) and another is mineral availability. If you are using a lot of protein supplements instead of actual dairy, this can mean that the minerals such as calcium and phosphorus are low. If overall intake is low, for whatever reason, the body will re-absorb calcium from the bones to maintain blood levels. Low bone mineral density will therefore make the bones more susceptible to breaks and they will take longer to heal.

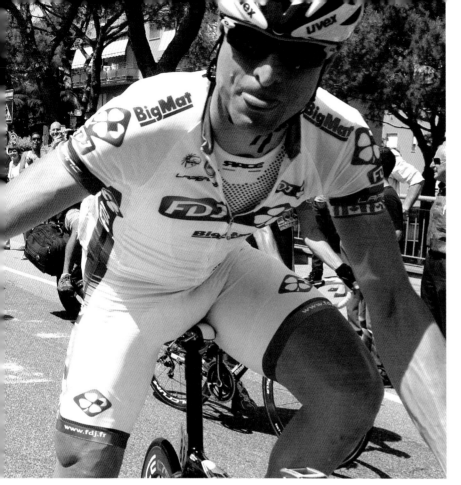

Keep a food diary

One of the most powerful weight management tools is to keep a simple food diary. The very act of recording what you eat makes you more aware of what you're putting in and less likely to reach for those extra couple of biscuits. Many people who have previously struggled with weight but didn't think they were overeating often find, once they keep a food diary, that a lot of food sneaks under the radar. A food diary will make you more aware of junk calories – a prime example being alcohol. Calories from alcohol are effectively 'empty calories', which tend to be stored almost immediately as fat. One of the simplest ways for many people to lose weight is to just cut out alcohol. You should also use your food diary to keep a tally of your calorie intake for the purpose of working out your energy balance. Remember, this needs to be continually reassessed and tweaked depending on how our weight and body composition is changing.

Only diet when you're healthy

Restricting energy intake and carrying on with training and racing puts a big strain on the body. If you've got a cold or are healing up after a crash, you shouldn't be trying to actively lose weight. You'll be compromising your immune system and potentially lengthening the time you have to spend off your bike. Another time that is stressful to the body is if you're travelling, especially considering you're likely to be upping your training too, so a training camp is not ideal for weight loss.

The importance of protein

Maintenance and protection of your lean muscle tissue is a real priority and the nutrient that provides this is quality protein. When I'm working with a rider who is trying to lose weight, the quality and amount of protein they receive is something we never compromise on. It's also vital to ensure they're getting enough of the good fats too. We'll predominately look at altering carbohydrate intake, reducing the amount they're consuming and matching its availability and timing to the riding they're doing. Both practical demonstrations and scientific research have shown that increasing protein helps to protect the muscle mass when on an energy-restricted diet. By all means cut back on calories and carbohydrates, but never cut back on quality protein.

Avoid faddy diets and processed weight-loss foods

You'll constantly read about the latest must-do diet for fast weight loss, but the reality is there's no shortcut or magic bullet. Even pro athletes get sucked into believing certain supplements help weight loss. I have lost count of the number of times a pro has asked me about the latest wonder product. Genuine fat loss, without losing lean tissue also, takes time, patience and discipline. Realistic sustainable fat loss is about 0.5 kg (1.1 lb) per week. If you're losing significantly more than this, it's likely to be lean tissue and water loss.

Steer clear of commercially available diet foods. They might be labelled as low-fat but are often packed with sugar. If you manage and prepare your own food and meals, you know exactly what you're getting.

Gym work

Another way you can protect your lean muscle mass while trying to lose fat is to include some resistance work in your training. This especially applies to riders who are over 30 because, without the stimulation of resistance training, ageing causes a progressive loss of lean mass. You don't have to necessarily hit the gym; doing some over geared or torque work on the bike has the same effect. Gym and big gear work can leave your legs feeling heavy and sore, so it's best left to out-of-season training blocks, which also fits in well with fat loss.

WEIGHT GAIN

When most riders are talking about gaining weight, they're talking about increasing their lean tissue mass. (I don't think I've ever heard of a rider wanting to gain fat!) A bigger cross-sectional area of muscle will deliver greater peak power. This is why track sprinters such as Sir Chris Hoy have such phenomenally huge legs. For endurance riders, this peak power isn't so important. The key figure for them is Functional Threshold Power (FTP), which is approximately the power they can sustain for an hour. Cross-sectional area of muscle has very little bearing on FTP, but the architecture and density of mitochondria within the muscle does. However, for a more all-round rider, the ability to sprint at the end of a criterium, punch up a short climb or close a gap does require a bit more top-end force, so you can't just be a diesel engine.

Especially if you're under-muscled, the idea behind putting on some lean mass is that both the mitochondrial density and peak power can be increased. You effectively become a bit of a hybrid, and track endurance riders, such as British track rider Ed Clancy, are great examples of this kind of athlete. His peak power isn't quite enough to be a world-class sprinter and his FTP won't make him a Grand Tour contender, but he's deadly in an omnium, team pursuit or a punchy circuit race.

For road pros, some lean weight gain can also improve their robustness, making them less prone to injuries. We'd be looking to increase their supporting musculature, such as their lower back, glutes and abdominals. This wouldn't necessarily increase their power output directly, but, at the end of a long race, it will help them to keep riding strongly. Read the example about Joe Dombrowski's Pro Story (page 155).

If you are looking to gain some lean mass, don't fall into the old mindset of thinking you have to massively up your calorie consumption. As long as you're eating well and providing adequate quality protein, approximately 2 g per kg of body weight, the key is providing the correct training stimuli and, for muscle gain, that's some gym work. More and more pro cyclists are now spending time in the gym and, by being stronger and less under-muscled, are definitely seeing the benefits in their riding and body composition.

Almost all amateur riders would benefit from including a couple of sessions of all-round strengthening work in their weekly routines. There can be a slight conflict during concurrent training, when you're trying to build strength/lean mass and endurance at the same time, but it can be managed with good training planning and nutrition. The secret is not necessarily pushing more and more protein, but eating good-quality protein and structuring it frequently around the day so that your muscles always have the amino acids they require available to them.

PRO STORY: JOE DOMBROWSKI

At the end of the 2015 season it was decided that Joe Dombrowski of the Cannondale/Drapac professional cycling team had a great engine, but needed to be stronger and increase his muscle mass. He underwent a programme of gym training with an emphasis on gaining muscle mass specifically around his glutes, lower back and quads. He gained about 4 kg (8.8 lb) of lean muscle mass. This shows that, although difficult, it's not impossible for an endurance athlete in a heavy conditioning phase to gain significant lean tissue. Both training and nutrition need to be carefully planned out in order to maximize gains and minimize the potential compromise to on-the-bike training and performance.

In the winter, Dombrowski's programme focused around three gym sessions a week. The plan was that these would be either on easy days or he would do the gym work later in the day after riding. This is because different types of training generate different stimuli for the muscles to adapt to. Endurance work tells the muscle to produce more mitochondria and strength work tells the muscle to make thicker muscle fibre. The length of time the body maintains the stimulus is affected by the intensity and frequency of the training. From a strength point of view the stimulus can last for over 24 hours, but can be blunted by endurance work during that period. So doing gym work first could be counterproductive to the gains achieved from it and could also have a detrimental effect on a subsequent cycling session. If you're looking to include some strength work in your training, you should bear this in mind. Try to schedule in the strength work at the end of the day or on days when you aren't training on the bike. Allow 48–72 hours between strength workouts and try to avoid high-intensity or long duration bike sessions in the 24 hours following them.

From a nutritional perspective, when I have a rider who is trying to increase muscle mass I will use certain supplements to help support the body. These would include about 5 g of creatine per day. I find this dose provides the benefits without causing the excessive weight gain from bloating that traditional loading protocols can lead to. Some additional leucine in the form of Branch

Chain Amino Acids (BCAA), approximately 2 g per day after the gym session can also help. Leucine has been shown to amplify the protein synthesis after resistance work, aiding both muscle growth and repair. I would also recommend fish oils or another omega-3 supplement. They're anti-inflammatory and can also help to maintain muscle mass. These and other supplements are discussed in greater detail in Chapter 9 (see pages 163–187). I would also tend to use a protein recovery drink, mainly because it is more convenient to have straight after training and the exact quantities can be more easily controlled. I would also advise some slow-release protein before bed; yoghurt or cottage cheese are ideal because they are a good source of casein proteins. These tend to be drip released into the body throughout the night which can also help the gain and maintenance of muscle mass. Even a hot chocolate made with about 300 ml of milk is a good option as we're not looking for a massive protein hit but something that will supply about 10–15 g of protein. By following this plan, Joe gained the muscle mass he needed and, in doing so, hit the 2016 season a stronger and more robust rider. He felt that during the 2016 Giro d'Italia he climbed better than he'd ever done before and put that down to the extra muscle he'd gained.

KNOWLEDGE TO TAKE AWAY

- **Think about your goals** Weight loss isn't an easy or a fast way to performance gains. Think about the type of riding you do and whether investing the time and energy in more focused and effective training may be more worthwhile.

- **Find out your body composition** The scales do lie so find a qualified professional to measure your skin folds and have them regularly retested. Ideally this should be on a monthly basis depending on goals.

- **Personalise your plan** Online calculators can provide a useful starting point for working out your calorific need and energy balance but cannot be relied upon. Use the results of your skin-fold tests to tweak your diet and training.

- **Time your fat loss** When you're training hard it's not a good time to try and lose fat. Also, avoid dieting when you're ill, recovering from an injury or travelling abroad.

- **Protect your lean mass** Losing lean mass equates to less power on the bike and the likelihood of long-term greater fat gain. Don't restrict calories too drastically, prioritise quality protein and consider including some resistance work in your training.

- **Don't look for faddy shortcuts** If a miracle diet sounds too good to be true, that's because it is. Avoid pre-packaged low-fat diet meals and stick to whole foods, healthy eating and fuelling your training.

- **Do not deprive yourself completely** If you like a bit of chocolate, then include a few squares of dark chocolate a day. This will give you your chocolate fix but keep the calories low.

TURKEY BURGERS

Packed with lean turkey mince, egg and quinoa, these burgers are a delicious protein feast. Have them in the fridge ready to cook when you get home or, as they're delicious cold, cook before you head out. Serve with a salad and some sweet potato wedges (see page 70) if you need some carbohydrates.

Servings 4 (4 large burgers)
Calories per serving: 180 kcal
Carbohydrate per serving: 5 g
Fat per serving: 2.7 g
Protein per serving: 35 g

INGREDIENTS

500 g minced turkey thigh
1 medium egg
30 g quinoa flakes
1 medium onion, chopped
1 garlic clove, crushed
1 tbsp olive oil
Salt and pepper, to taste

METHOD

1. Prepare the burgers 1–2 hours before you intend to cook them.

2. In a frying pan, heat the olive oil over a medium heat. Add the onion and garlic and cook for 5–10 minutes or until soft. Remove from pan and transfer into a large mixing bowl and allow to thoroughly cool.

3. Add all of the other ingredients to the mixing bowl and, using your hands, thoroughly mix and shape into four equal-sized burgers.

4. Place the burgers on a plate, cover in clingfilm and place in the fridge for 1–2 hours to firm up.

5. Preheat your oven to 180 °C (Gas 4).

6. Bake the burgers on a non-stick baking tray for 20–25 minutes, turning once. Serve with a green salad with a Balsamic dressing (optional).

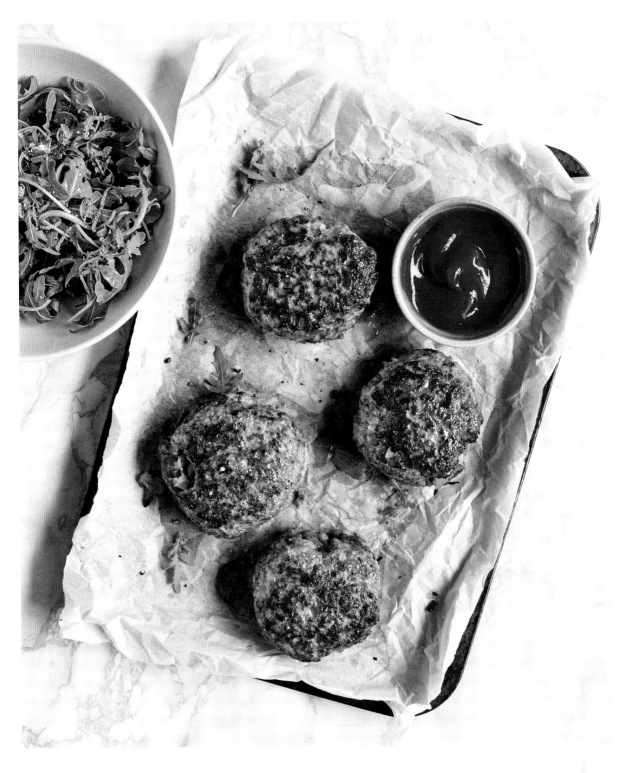

CAPRESE SALAD

···

This is a real cyclists' favourite. It's ideal as a light post-ride snack in the summer as it's quick to make, refreshing and delivers a decent amount of protein. Tomatoes are also high in lycopene, a powerful antioxidant. It's also a good option as a dinner-party starter with this amount being ideal for two. I've used low-fat mozzarella just to keep the calories down, but if you're not trying to lose weight, opt for full-fat.

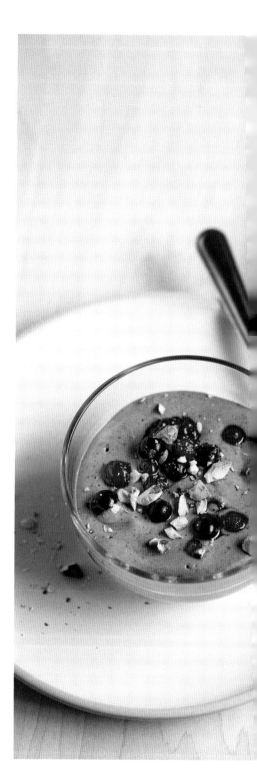

Serves 1
Calories per serving:
    283 kcal
Carbohydrate per serving:
    6 g
Fat per serving: 17.4 g
Protein per serving: 25 g

INGREDIENTS
1 fresh, low-fat mozzarella
    ball
1 medium tomato
A few fresh basil leaves
Drizzle of olive oil
Drizzle of Balsamic
    vinegar
Salt and pepper, to taste

METHOD

1. Slice the cheese and tomato and arrange in layers on a plate.

2. Finish with the basil and dress with a light drizzle of the oil and vinegar and season with salt and pepper.

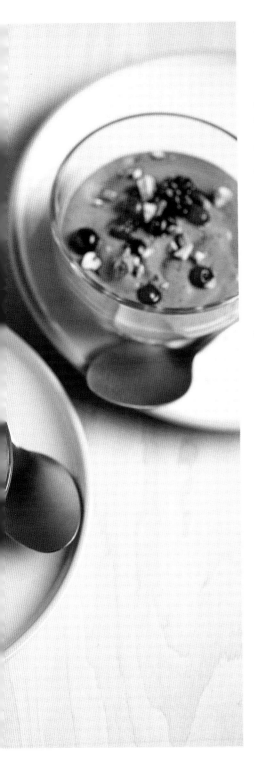

VERY BERRY PROTEIN FLUFF

. . . .

Protein fluff, so-called because it's like a fluffy mousse, has been popular in strength sports for some time as it's a great way to get a dessert fix without the sugar and with a big protein hit. I developed this recipe for Olympic, World and Commonwealth track cycling champion Victoria Pendleton as part of her 2012 London Olympic Games preparation. It also includes milled flaxseed, which is high in omega-3 oils. You can use any protein powder, but if you use a flavoured one then a subtle flavour such as vanilla works best.

Serves 2
Calories per serving:
 204 kcal
Carbohydrate per serving:
 8 g
Fat per serving: 9 g
Protein per serving: 20 g

INGREDIENTS
2–3 tbsp protein powder
125 g frozen mixed
 berries, thawed
100 ml skimmed milk
30 g milled flaxseed
Handful of pistachios,
 chopped

METHOD

1. Place all of the ingredients, reserving a few berries for the top, into a food processor and blend for a few minutes to get plenty of air into it.

2. Serve into bowls and sprinkle with a few chopped pistachios and berries. Serve chilled.

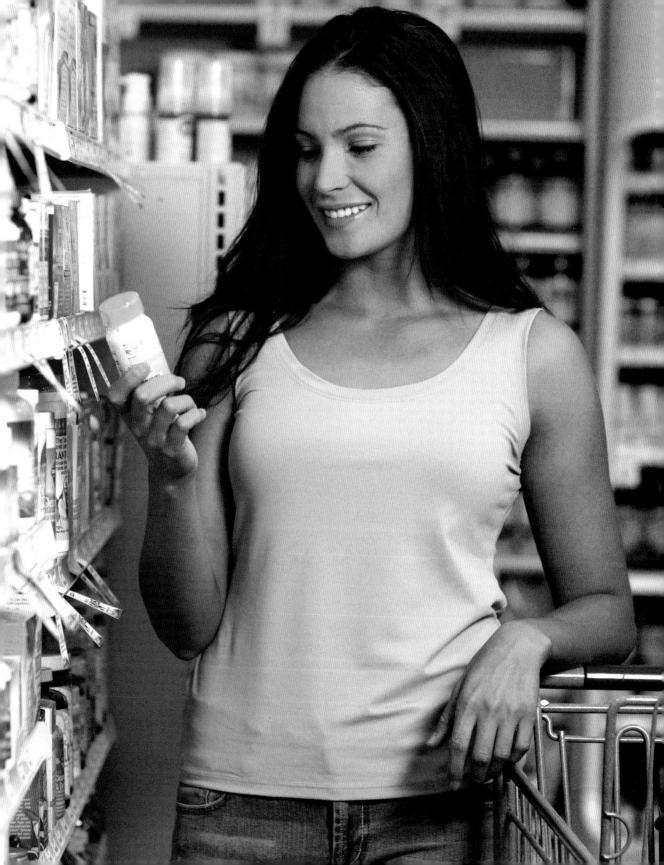

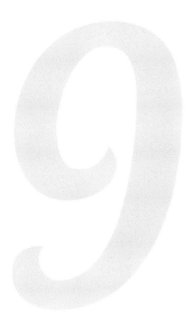

SUPPLEMENTS

A dietary supplement is simply an addition to your normal diet
that is intended to provide nutrients that may otherwise not be consumed in sufficient quantities. Based on this definition, you could argue that a gel is a supplement as it's supplying additional carbohydrates. The way I look at it though is to split products into sports foods and supplements. Sports foods are the products that supply the macronutrients in a way that is more convenient and in a more controlled format. For example, an energy bar or gel provides the same carbohydrate and energy as a banana, but is more practical to carry in your jersey pocket on a long ride. A protein recovery drink provides the same as milk and a banana, but again is more convenient and easy to use. Supplements, on the other hand, are really the nutrients that can be difficult to get from your diet or may improve performance.

From a sports perspective, supplements that improve your performance are said to be ergogenic. Cyclists are always on the lookout for the next super supplement and there are plenty of manufacturers looking to relieve them of their hard-earned money with promises of extra power, improved endurance, fat loss and guaranteed personal bests. However, at best the gains from supplements will be marginal and many are simply snake oil. Before looking for magic bullets to improve your cycling, make sure you've got all the basics right. Follow the nutritional advice in this book, use a structured training plan and make sure your position on the bike is correct. For the pros who'll have ticked all these boxes, it might be a case of accumulating marginal gains, but for most amateurs, it's a case of first minimising maximal losses! There is a real culture in sport, at all levels, of using supplements. I work hard to try and educate athletes about appropriate supplement use, but no matter what I say, there is still a tendency for athletes to look for the next miracle supplement. On reflection I have only worked with one Olympian who did not use any nutritional supplements and that was Amir Kahn, the British boxer who won a silver medal at the 2004 Athens Olympic games.

STUDYING SUPPLEMENTS

One of the problems with evaluating many supplements is that the research is often incomplete when it comes to enhancing sports performance at an elite level. Many substances should in theory boost performance and, indeed, when tested on animals in the laboratory, do yield promising results; however, just because something allows a mouse to run for longer doesn't mean it'll do the same for you on your bike! The next stage – testing on humans – is fraught with difficulties. Once all the ethical constraints have been negotiated, researchers have then got to find subjects and this is one of the biggest hurdles to overcome. Most studies are performed on sedentary subjects or, at best, keen amateurs. No top-level sportsperson is going to risk taking an unproven substance so obtaining meaningful data is incredibly difficult. There are no shortcuts or magic bullets I can offer you, I'm afraid, and performance boils down to talent, smart consistent training and sound nutrition. Legally, there are very few ergogenic aids that have any real value and, at the elite level, I'm yet to be 100 per cent convinced of any. Be extremely suspicious of claims of performance gains and remember, if you're competing, ignorance or a tainted supplement are no excuses for a failed dope test.

COMMON CYCLING SUPPLEMENTS

Though we've already discussed a few specific supplements in earlier chapters, let's revisit them along, with a few more that are popular among cyclists.

Protein

Although probably falling under my sports food definition, I'm often asked about consuming supplementary protein in the form of protein powders and whether they're necessary or a waste of money.

A male cyclist will typically require 1.2–1.6 g/kg/day of protein, with female riders requiring about 15 per cent less (0.9–1.2 g/kg/day). For an 80-kg male cyclist, this translates to 96–128 g of protein, which could be provided by:

Three egg omelette ....18 g
Handful of pistachios..5 g
Tuna sandwich with 120 g can tuna..........................27 g
Cottage cheese, 120 g ....8 g
Two turkey breast steaks...43 g
500 ml whole milk..16 g
Total ....127 g

A 60-kg female cyclist would need 54–72 g of protein, which could be provided by:

Two egg omelette ....12 g
Handful of pistachios..5 g
Tuna sandwich, with half a drained can ....13.5 g
Cottage cheese, half tbsp...7 g
One turkey breast steak ....21.5 g
250 ml whole milk..8 g
Total ....68 g

As you can see, even hitting the upper end of the range doesn't require huge amounts. This doesn't mean that there's no place for protein powders. They can provide a convenient and controlled way to ensure you're getting the nutrients you need; for example, immediately after a ride or as you're cooling down on your ride home, sipping on a protein drink is by far the easiest way to start your recovery.

Health and well-being supplements

There are a multitude of products aimed at keeping you healthy and protecting the body, rather than directly improving your cycling performance. Many are based on some evidence and many people really find they get genuine benefit from them.

GLUCOSAMINE

Glucosamine is an amino sugar that is normally produced from crustacean shells and therefore shouldn't be taken by anyone with shellfish allergies. It is marketed to support the structure and function of joints, however, although laboratory studies were promising, clinical tests have been less convincing. That said, many people who suffer from aching joints find its mild anti-inflammatory effects to be beneficial. It is often associated with older people, but I have known professional cyclists use it as part of general rehabilitation following a bone break in a crash. Clinical studies have shown a dose of 1500 mg/day to be safe, but this shouldn't be exceeded.

ANTIOXIDANTS

Antioxidant-type products, which include ingredients like green tea extract, super fruit juices and certain vitamins, are designed to help the body deal with the supposedly damaging free radicals produced during metabolic processes. Free radicals are atoms or groups of atoms with an odd (unpaired) number of electrons and can be formed when oxygen interacts with certain molecules. Once formed, these highly reactive radicals can start a chain reaction, like dominoes. Their chief danger comes from the damage they can do when they react with important cellular components such as DNA or the cell membrane. Cells may function poorly or die if this occurs. To prevent free-radical damage, therefore, the body has a defence system of antioxidants. The idea behind talking antioxidant supplements is that, because we produce more free radicals when our bodies work harder, antioxidant products reduce the impact of the increased amount of free radicals. If you're eating plenty of brightly coloured fruit and vegetables and ensuring you get those 'glow nutrients', there shouldn't be any need to supplement antioxidant intake. However, if you're training especially hard, under stress or unable to obtain fresh fruit and vegetables, you may want to consider a supplement. A popular and potent antioxidant source is the tart juice from the Montmorency cherry. This is available as a juice, in gels and as capsules. I regularly use Montmorency with riders when they are in really hard training or competition. There are a host of antioxidant products available – one I commonly use with riders, which you could try, contains green tea and pine bark extract – and they all serve the same function.

Multivitamins and multi-minerals

These are probably the most common of all supplements used by both athletes and non-athletes, but under normal conditions with a good balanced diet, there is little need for them. However, many athletes like to have a safety blanket and feel that taking a multivitamin will ensure that they're getting what they need and covering their bases. It is rare that I advise athletes to take one, but if they do want to, I like to use a product that provides a broad spectrum of the vitamins and minerals and does not supply above the 100 per cent RDA levels. There's no point in exceeding these levels and it could even be dangerous. Excess water-soluble vitamins, such as vitamin C, will simply be excreted, but fat-soluble vitamins, such as A, D, E and K, can build up to toxic levels in the body. If you're also taking other supplements, it's important to check that you're not doubling up on any doses.

IRON

As previously discussed iron can be an issue for endurance athletes (see page 20). A lot of people have lower levels of iron stores and this can be for a number of reasons, including diet and lifestyle compromising absorption: tea, coffee and antacids, for example, can all reduce our iron absorption; and female athletes can also suffer low iron levels due to heavy menstrual bleeding (see page 207). There are many iron products on the market but, even if you

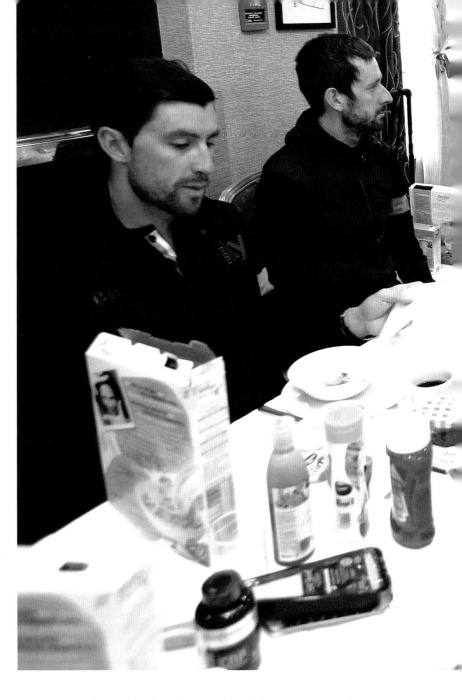

suspect you have low levels, you shouldn't just start taking one. Some people are very sensitive to iron supplements in that they can cause stomach problems. If you are suffering from unusual fatigue or poor recovery, my recommendation is to have a blood

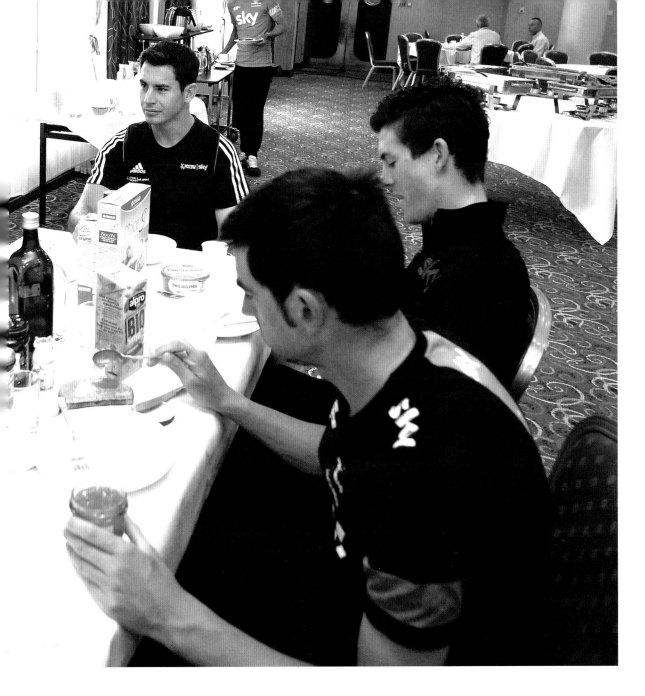

test for iron stores and then seek professional advice. A lot of the multivitamin and multi-mineral products will contain about 15 mg of iron and that should be sufficient for most people.

VITAMIN D

We've discussed vitamin D and its importance for bone health (see page 20), but it also has a number of other key roles in the body, including supporting immunity. In recent years we have gained a greater understanding regarding its role. Modern research has shown that many people have inadequate levels of vitamin D, especially in the Northern Hemisphere during the winter, which can affect recovery and general well-being. A blood test is the only way to confirm your levels. However, this is quite expensive to do privately, but if you present your doctor with fatigue in the winter months, they should run a blood test for you. There are also now companies which offer DIY pin-prick tests which can be sent off for analysis. However, for a lot of people, taking a prophylactic dose in the winter can be a good idea. The current upper dosage of vitamin D that an individual should take, unless under medical care, is 400 iu (100 mg) per day.

Omega-3 oils (eicosapentaenoic acid)

A large proportion of the UK population regularly takes some form of fish oil, mostly cheap cod liver oil, but many have little idea of why they're taking it. I brought the idea of using fish oil into sport from my clinical work in hospitals. Cancer patients suffer from a stress-related muscle wastage, known as cachexia, which has no relation to calorie deficit: even if they're eating enough, it still happens. Fish oils, or more specifically, the omega-3 fatty acid eicosapentaenoic acid (EPA), help prevents it from happening and aids the retention of lean tissue. Hard training or racing is a similar stress on the body and omega-3 can perform the same function. Omega-3 fats are not only linked to reducing inflammation, but also positively influencing blood vessels and protein synthesis. If your normal diet is high in omega-3, containing lots of oily fish and seeds, you could be getting enough, but it's the ratio with omega-6 that's important.

Due to the high proportion of processed vegetable oils in

modern diets, which are very rich in omega-6, the levels in our bodies tend to be disproportionally high. It has been suggested that an ideal ratio would be 1:1 whereas, for many people, it is 1:20. Try to reduce your omega-6 intake; cooking with olive or coconut oil rather than sunflower oil will help massively. You can also positively improve your omega-3 intake by including regular oily fish and milled flaxseed in your diet. Incidentally, although we can get omega-3 from oily fish, the fish themselves obtain it from the krill and algae which they consume.

For many people, including athletes in hard training, a supplement is definitely useful. You have to ensure, however, you're taking a high-quality oil with at least 60 per cent omega-3 and which will deliver 2 g of EPA daily. With high-dose omega-3 capsules, this may be between three and five capsules a day. Cheap cod liver oils just won't do.

Probiotics and prebiotics

We spoke about the function of pro and prebiotics in Chapter 2 (see pages 27–28 and 34–36). Prebiotics are the food which the good bacteria (probiotics) use. These bacteria are essential for gut health and good digestion. Prebiotics are mainly indigestible carbohydrate, in other words, fibre. The main active types are inulin and fructooligosaccharides (FOS), which are commonly found in whole grains, onions, bananas, garlic, leeks, artichokes and fortified foods (foods which have an ingredient added for health benefits). You can also buy both inulin and FOS supplements, but with a balanced diet, they shouldn't be necessary.

The bacteria (probiotics) are your gut flora and are believed to help support the immune system by protecting the micro villi, the small, finger-like projections in your gut (see page 27). The current school of thought is to include a variety of different cultures of probiotics which will introduce a mix of species of bacteria. The two main types of product available are capsules and 'live' cultures. Neither one is more beneficial than the other, but the capsules are more convenient for travelling. With the capsules the probiotics are generally freeze-dried, which puts them into a dormant state, and are then reactivated when consumed. The live probiotics are usually in fermented products such as Actimel or Yakult. Kefir, a traditional culture from the Caucasus Mountains, which is growing in popularity, is effectively a DYI probiotic culture (see page 36). Pickled foods, such as sauerkraut, can also help to support probiotic function. There is generally no need to constantly take probiotics, but if you have had a digestive upset, are travelling abroad or have taken antibiotics, which will have killed your beneficial gut bacteria along with the harmful bacteria, they can be beneficial.

Colostrum

Colostrum is the first milk produced by mammals and the commercially available version used as a supplement is bovine (cow) colostrum. However, as it's vital for a calf's health to have the true 'first milk', what we end up with is actually the milk produced after the first 12 hours following the birth of a calf. Colostrum is high in growth factors that help to protect the micro villi of the intestines, and there is reasonable scientific data to suggest that it is protective to the gut, especially when exercising in the heat (see page 27).

Energised greens

These are a relatively new type of product which by my own definition could probably be categorised as a sports food rather than a supplement. They combine different green (high chlorophyll) vegetable sources, such as spinach, broccoli and spirulina, which are freeze-dried and powdered. This results in a highly concentrated vegetable powder. As you can imagine getting the taste right with these products can be a real challenge and the majority of them do taste a bit like pond water. However, manufacturers have worked hard to include natural flavourings and stevia, a natural sweetener, to create more palatable products. The main idea behind these products is that they are naturally alkaline so they can help with the alkalinity of the gut, aiding digestion and gut health. I'll also use them with riders as part of the gut rehab plan (see pages 33–34) as a way to ensure that they're getting their 'glow nutrients' and fibre without the gut-stressing bulk of whole vegetables and salads.

Glutamine

Glutamine is one of the most abundant amino acids and it plays a key role in gut health and the immune system. It works by being a key component of glutathione, which is an important antioxidant for the body. It has been used in intensive care and burns units to help support critically ill patients. At times of high stress, some athletes have found benefits taking between 5–20 g per day in either capsule or powder form.

Ergogenic supplements

These are the supplements that can supposedly improve your performance on the bike, tolerance to training and racing and your ability to recover. There are literally hundreds of substances with claimed performance benefits and you could easily write a whole book dedicated to analysing their use and effiancy alone. However, the ones listed below are those which I have worked with and believe to be worth considering. However, any performance boosts you do get will be marginal at best and, for the vast majority of riders, investing their time and money in optimising training, nutrition and bike set-up will result in far more measurable gains.

CAFFEINE

Although enhanced fat mobilisation is often touted as being the reason for performance gains with caffeine, its main benefit, when

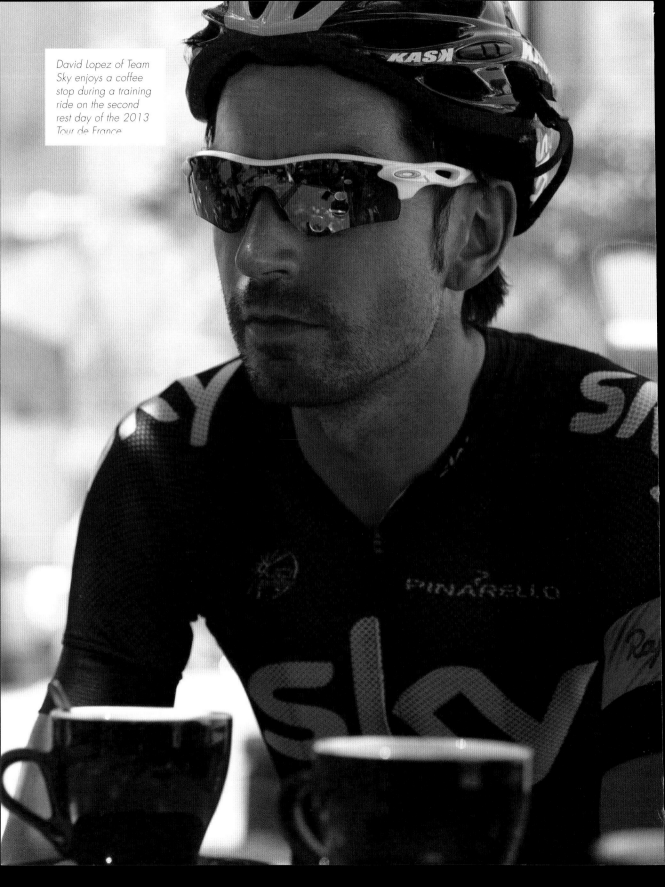

David Lopez of Team Sky enjoys a coffee stop during a training ride on the second rest day of the 2013 Tour de France

taken in conjunction with some sugar, is to give you a neurological lift. This can either be before a hard effort, such as a time trial when a rider would take a caffeinated gel during their warm-up, or near the end of a long ride when they need a bit of a boost. Studies have shown that a dose of 3–6 mg/kg is required for a performance boost. A typical 250 ml cup of brewed coffee will contain 115 mg of caffeine and an espresso shot 75 mg, but exact amounts can vary massively. I don't recommend any sort of loading protocols though and we are always really aware on stage races that excessive caffeine can lead to anxiety and poor sleep. It's also worth noting that you do become habituated to caffeine, so, to gain any ergogenic benefits, if you're a regular coffee drinker, you may need to taper your intake prior to key events. A two-week taper, where you gradually reduce intake during the first week and completely abstain during the second, is probably best. If you tend to consume a fair amount of coffee, you might find you suffer headaches for four to five days if you try to go cold turkey so a more gradual approach, maybe halving intake each day during the first week, is sensible.

Buffers

The harder we exercise the greater the demand for oxygen. Above a certain intensity, the energy demand increases and outstrips available oxygen supply. We produce more energy anaerobically (i.e. without oxygen). The consequence of this anaerobic, energy-production pathway is that we produce lactate. Many people think that lactate is bad, but in fact it is a very useful metabolic substance for the body and is recycled for energy. The downside with the lactate produced is that we also get hydrogen ions – in other words, acid. This leads to a state of acidosis in the body and is responsible for the burning-legs sensation you feel during a hard effort on the bike and a slowing down of the breakdown of carbohydrates into energy.

Buffers work by neutralising the hydrogen ions, delaying the burn and allowing you to go a bit harder for a bit longer. We can think about the buffers within the muscle cell and those outside it: the most well-known buffer supplement is probably sodium bicarbonate, which neutralises some of the acid as it migrates out of the cell; inside the cell the main buffers are protein based and include creatine and carnosine (made up of beta alanine and histodine).

SODIUM BICARBONATE

Simple baking soda that you find in your kitchen cupboard buffers acid build-up and might also improve tolerance to heat due to plasma expansion, increasing the liquid content of your blood. I've used it with team pursuit riders and there are some decent studies which seem to support its use, but I'm not 100 per cent convinced whether it does give measurable benefits to elite athletes. However, it seems to be part of the culture and the riders like it, so they take it as much for the placebo boost and pre-race ritual as anything else. If you do decide to try it though, practise beforehand as the gastric side effects can be – well – explosive, and you don't want to ruin an expensive skin-suit! I suggest a lower dose than you often see recommended of 0.2 g/kg, which you should take dissolved in 500 ml of water or juice about one and half hours before riding. If you find it useful, it can be used as a training aid for repeated threshold sessions. It can help riders recover between efforts and improve the training quality, which can lead to an improved training effect.

BETA-ALANINE

Beta-alanine is one of the non-essential amino acids. A very prominent sports scientist, Dr Roger Harris from the University of Wales Aberystwyth, who was responsible for discovering the potential benefits of creatine, studied the muscle buffer carnosine. He discovered that the limiting factor to carnosine levels in the body was the availability of one of its component parts, beta-alanine. He found that, by increasing beta-alanine in the diet, you could increase the carnosine and improve the buffering in the muscle. Initially it was difficult to find the isolated amino acid, so athletes consumed foods, such as turkey, which was known to be high in it. I first used it with speed skaters, using a combination of food and supplements, including my Turkey Power Soup recipe (see page 185). Now it's easily available as a supplement. It takes about four weeks of taking about 4 g a day of beta-alanine to load the system and it can then be maintained on about 1 g a day. This is a very popular supplement with cyclists, but I see it more as a training aid than a competition boost. If you are doing high-intensity workouts with multiple sprint or supra-threshold efforts, it can help you push that bit harder and achieve more during the session. Many riders do, however, experience a tingling sensation after consuming beta-alanine. This is completely harmless and it could be argued that this tangible physiological effect of taking the supplement increases its efficacy due to an enhanced placebo effect.

CREATINE

Creatine is an interesting compound which is similar in structure to the amino acids, the building blocks of proteins. From a performance point of view, it helps in the explosive phase of exercise when the predominant energy source is phosphocreatine. Increasing the stores enables the body to perform better in repeated sprints, in effect reducing your fatigue and enabling back-to-back top-end efforts. It is also a buffer, but that is not the primary use as a nutritional supplement.

If you search for creatine dosage on the internet, you will find lots of protocols recommending a loading phase followed by a maintenance phase. The traditional recommendation is to have a loading phase of 20 g a day for a week to 10 days. However, this can cause bloating and a weight gain of as much as 2 kg.

This is primarily because, as the muscle absorbs the creatine, it also stores water and swells the size of the muscles. This, combined with its benefits for explosive movements, is why it's so popular with athletes involved in strength, power and contact sports. For cyclists, it can definitely be a help during strength and muscle-building phases of training and I've been using it with team pursuit riders for a number of years. However, to avoid the weight gain and bloating, I tend to avoid a loading phase and favour a relatively low dose of 5 g/day.

NITRATES

To most people this means beetroot juice, which has become incredibly popular, with claims of both health benefits and enhanced endurance sports performance. It's the nitrates in the beetroot that give rise to the effects and they're also found in strawberries and most leafy and root vegetables. When we eat nitrates, bacteria in our saliva convert about 20 per cent of it into nitrites. This is then absorbed and reduced to nitric oxide. This has a vasodilatory effect, increasing the size of blood vessels – an effect which can reduce blood pressure, improve oxygen transfer to muscle and potentially enhance some aspects of aerobic exercise performance. There have been a number of studies showing improved performance in previously sedentary and low-level athletes, but they haven't been replicated with elite-level performers. If you do want to try it before a sportive or long training ride, it certainly won't do any harm, but be prepared for alarmingly pink urine and faeces. Although I haven't used it specifically with pro riders because of its lack of proven effect on elite athletes, many of the juices I make do contain beetroot for its high vitamin and mineral content. The riders certainly find the brightly coloured urine an amusing side effect. The dosage is estimated to be about 500 ml of juice or approximately 750 g of beetroot before juicing, taken a few hours before exercise. You can buy concentrated shots as well and nitrate-containing gels.

BCAAS

These branched chain amino acids – leucine, isoleucine and valine – are a special group that are differentiated from the other amino acids by their structure. They have been linked to helping to prevent central nervous system fatigue in endurance exercise and more recently leucine has been shown to increase protein synthesis after exercise, building and repairing muscle. Be aware though that these are 'molecular' laboratory-based studies that are looking at the gene expression, i.e. switching on the genes that tell the muscle to increase the protein synthesis. Whey protein is already high in BCAAs, but supplementation is popular with many riders at a dosage of between 2–5 g daily. I work with riders who love to use them, but suspect that the benefits they feel are largely psychological. I do not tend to recommend them as the riders I work with will be getting plenty from the high-quality protein they're already consuming.

L-CARNITINE

This is the amino acid that is used to shuttle fat in the cell into the mitochondria, the powerhouses of the cell. It is believed that the carnitine is a limiting factor in fat oxidation and studies have shown that, by increasing the muscle carnitine level, fat oxidation and weight loss can be enhanced. The leap of faith for a practical application of these findings is that taking extra carnitine in your diet actually increases the carnitine level in the muscle cells. Well-controlled studies have shown that you can do this, but it takes a long time to build up the carnitine levels and that you need to take a lot of extra carbohydrates to support the absorption into the muscle, which would probably offset any weight-loss benefits. In saying all of that, a lot of professional riders do love to take gels containing carnitine. Again, it's the belief they're taking something of benefit that probably gives them a bit of a boost.

Quality Assurance

When considering any nutritional products or supplements, the issues of quality assurance and contamination should be at the forefront of any athlete's mind. Currently the nutrition products industry is fairly unregulated so you have to rely on the honesty and integrity of the companies and your own scrutiny. A massive part of my role when dealing with elite athletes is ensuring the quality of any products they're taking. There are two main aspects to this: the first is ensuring that the products contain what they say they do and in sufficient amounts to have the desired effect; the second is that they don't contain any unwanted ingredients or contaminants. This includes substances that could lead to failing a dope test.

Under the code of the World Anti-Doping Agency (WADA), the athlete takes full responsibility for what they put into their body. This is termed 'strict liability'. So, if they fail a test because of a contaminated supplement, that's no excuse and full sanctions will be taken. There have been many cases of top-level athletes being caught out in this way and receiving a doping violation. This can happen very easily as, in a lot of factories where nutritional products are made, they also make substances that contain these banned, but not illegal, contaminates. My job will therefore involve visiting the factory to ensure the risk of contamination is minimised and arranging batch testing by an independent laboratory to check that none has occurred. Nutritional companies that are supplying products to top teams and athletes will put multiple levels of protection in place. Along with batch testing, they'll retain samples of each batch for several years past their use-by date just in case there's a problem with it. Within the factory, security will be super-high, with the batches of products under CCTV surveillance from when they're on the production line to the point of delivery.

If you're competing at National level or Masters competition, there is a chance you could be drug tested. In theory, any rider with a UK racing licence can also be tested at any time, especially if there's suspicion about their results, and the same applies to

USA Cycling race license holders. You're responsible for ensuring that any supplements you may take are clean. The simplest way to do this and identify products that have been screened is to look for the Informed Choice logo. Informed Choice is a quality assurance programme for sports nutrition products, suppliers to the sports nutrition industry and supplement manufacturing facilities. The programme certifies that all nutritional supplements and/or ingredients have been tested for banned substances by the world-class sports anti-doping lab, LGC. This doesn't 100 per cent guarantee that the products don't contain contaminants, but it does reduce the risk. It would also demonstrate to WADA that you'd displayed due diligence.

Ketones: the supplement of the future

In Chapter 8 I mentioned ketones and how they may have performance-boosting value. It's worth highlighting them again as I think over the next few years we'll see them developed and commercially available. Sports scientists have already been exploring the possibility of using ketones to support exercise performance. Ketones are a naturally occurring range of chemicals produced by the body when it breaks down fat. The theory behind their use is that, by ingesting ketones, they will potentially provide an additional fuel source. We know that in hard exercise the body uses mainly carbohydrate and, if these supplies run low, this can be a limiting factor to performance. Acting as an additional fuel source, ketones would help to reduce glycogen depletion. By helping to conserve muscle carbohydrate stores, it would also help to feed the brain and reduce the chance of bonking. Studies have been promising and there's no doubt they have been used in professional sport. As previously mentioned though, the taste, the gastric distress they cause and cost (rumoured to be £2000 per litre), don't expect to be fuelling up on them anytime soon. However, watch this space, as they're an ergogenic supplement that could genuinely deliver a performance boost.

PRO STORY: SUBSTITUTING EPO FOR EPA

There is probably no other sporting event that's harder or more demanding of an athlete than a three-week Grand Tour. This is one of the main reasons why the use of injections, drips and illegal performance-enhancing drugs was so endemic. There was a mindset among the riders and support staff that, without them, completing, let alone battling for a win in, such a gruelling event was impossible. This created the doping arms race, culminating in widespread use of Erythropoietin (EPO) and blood doping, that the sport is only just now recovering from.

One of the most progressive changes in cycling was in 2011 when the UCI banned the use of intravenous recovery. Intravenous recovery was never doping, but was certainly on the grey side and represented the start of a slippery slope to more sinister and illegal practices.

To ride a Grand Tour clean, nutrition is key and, because of the unparalleled stress that's put on the riders, supplements play a large role. On one level, it's about supporting health and recovery. On the other, from the riders' emotional and psychological point of view, it gives a reassurance that there's something extra to help them perform because they know that a Grand Tour is going to push them beyond anything they do in training or in any other race.

Right from when I first began working on Grand Tours in the early 2000s, we began to look at nutritional protective packages to put in place around the riders. One of the key components of these protective packages was omega-3 fats. This was well before they became popular or even especially known to professional or elite athletes. We ensured they were receiving 2 g/day of eicosapentaenoic acid (EPA) and this really helped their bodies to deal with the demands of the race.

In the early 2000s, some of the young British talent were starting to break through from track to the road: two of these riders were the young Sir Bradley Wiggins and Steve Cummings. Even though we were not working directly with their pro teams, British Cycling was still providing remote support, based around some of the same principals we were using with the Great Britain Cycling Team track riders. I was tasked to provide nutrition support to help them cope with and manage with demanding Grand Tours. We prioritized them taking a good protein product straight after finishing a stage to aid recovery and, although this is commonplace now, it was revolutionary then.

From my hospital work, I had identified some of the clinical supplements that could be beneficial. One of these was a protein/energy supplement that was fortified with EPA. This was designed for patients suffering with cachexia (weight loss associated with cancer), but seemed perfect to use with our aspiring pro riders. The product provided 2 g of EPA, 20 g of protein and a total of about 400 kcal, it was the ideal recovery product. I have always wanted to develop something similar commercially, but cost has been prohibitive. However, by using a protein drink after your long rides in combination with EPA, you can mimic its effects.

In 2010, at Team Sky, we developed the idea of a nutritional protective package further. We weren't looking for or using supplements to directly boost the riders' performance, but were looking for ways, by improving their health, to allow them to keep performing right through to the end of the race.

The riders take a standard general multivitamin – not a super-high dose, just enough to cover the recommended daily amounts. This is a belt-and-braces approach that gives them a psychological reassurance too. They also take a small iron supplement because, when they're riding so long and so hard, there's a far higher turnover of iron and absorption is compromised too. They also have a general health and immunity product which contains ingredients such as green tea extract, that acts as a powerful antioxidant. This helps combat stress and aids recovery. The final product in the pack is of course the omega-3 oils capsules.

I make up packs for the riders that are distributed at the start of the race. The packs are divided into daily doses and include explanations of what the rider is taking, when they should take it and why. When combined with the amazing food provided by the team chef, we've found this approach to work well and have seen riders thrive in the final week of a Grand Tour. We've had riders come from other teams who having always struggled in the third week, find that they're now able to perform.

KNOWLEDGE TO TAKE AWAY

- **Sports foods vs supplements** *Sports foods, such as whey powders, gels and energy bars, provide macronutrients (carbohydrate, fat and protein) in a more convenient form than regular food. Supplements provide nutrients that may be hard to get in your diet, or are difficult to obtain in sufficient quantities, and may also have performance benefits.*

- **No shortcuts** *No supplement is a magic bullet to improved performance. You're always better off spending your time and money on training, bike set-up and optimum nutrition.*

- **Health and well-being vs ergogenic** *Some supplements, including multivitamins, iron and fish oils, enhance your health and recovery, rather than directly improve your cycling, whereas ergogenic supplements are performance enhancing.*

- **Quality Assurance and Informed Choice** *Whether you're a Tour de France rider or riding a local time trial, you're responsible for what you put in your body. Look for the Quality Assured or Informed Choice logo on any supplements you take.*

- **Eicosapentaenoic acid (EPA)** *If there's one supplement that I'd advise all riders to take, it's EPA-containing fish oils. I've seen the benefits in both a clinical and sporting environment. It won't make you ride faster but it'll help keep you healthy when training hard due to its anti-inflammatory and lean-muscle-mass preserving qualities. Don't worry if you're vegetarian or vegan as there are options for you (see pages 192–193).*

TURKEY POWER SOUP

High in the acid-buffering amino acid beta-alanine, this is also delicious, warming and high in quality protein. It's brilliant after a long winter's ride! This recipe makes five to six servings and extra portions can easily be frozen. Eat with some crusty bread to add carbohydrate, as required.

Serves 5–6
Calories per serving:
    342 kcal
Carbohydrate per serving: 12 g
Fat per serving: 7 g
Protein per serving: 50 g

INGREDIENTS

1 tbsp olive oil
1 kg turkey, diced
1 large onion, sliced
2 vegetable stock cubes
1 litre of water
1 large carrot, peeled and
    sliced
1 medium potato, peeled and
    diced
1 fillet smoked mackerel, skin
    removed
½ medium avocado, pitted
    and chopped
100 g quinoa, cooked
2 medium tomatoes, chopped
½ pepper, chopped

METHOD

1. In a frying pan, sauté the onion in the olive oil until softened.

2. Stir in the turkey and cook until browned.

3. Pour in the water and crumble the stock cubes. Add the carrot and potato and simmer for 20–30 minutes until the vegetables are softened.

4. Leave to cool, then add the remaining ingredients and liquidise.

5. Reheat to serve.

This recipe can also easily be made in the slow cooker. Follow the first three steps and then place in the slow cooker and cook according to the manufacturer's recommendations. Then follow the rest of the recipe as above.

BEETROOT JUICE

....

Whether you buy into the performance-boosting properties of beetroot or not, this juice is great for getting some 'glow nutrients' in and it's surprisingly delicious. If you are after the nitrates, a serving of this size will give you the prescribed dose. The beetroot should be raw for this recipe.

Serves 1
Calories per serving: 282 kcal
Carbohydrate per serving: 61 g
Fat per serving: 1 g
Protein per serving: 5.7 g

INGREDIENTS

750 g beetroot
   (or 500ml beetroot juice)
Small thumbnail fresh ginger
1 large apple
¼ cucumber

METHOD

1. Peel, core and chop the fruit and vegetables to suit your juicer.

2. Then simply juice and serve.

I recommend a juicer that separates the hard fibre from the juice. There are many on the market, but the slow juicers seem to extract more of the juice.

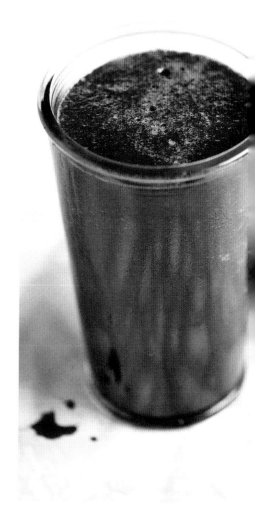

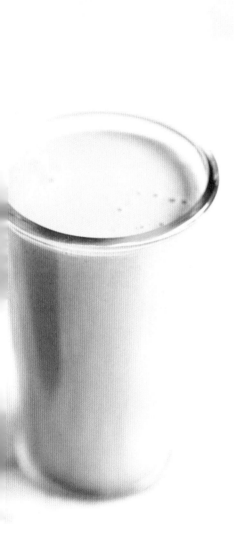

SUPER-GREEN SMOOTHIE

Something this colour must be good for you! It's full of 'glow nutrients' and easy-on-the-stomach soluble fibre for your friendly bacteria, and you'll also get a good serving of protein from the yoghurt. You can substitute kale instead of spinach in this recipe.

Serves 1
Calories per serving: 126 kcal
Carbohydrate per serving: 12.8 g
Fat per serving: 0.6 g
Protein per serving: 15 g

INGREDIENTS

150 g low-fat Greek yoghurt
½ carrot, peeled and chopped
75 g strawberries
Handful of fresh spinach, washed
Apple juice or water (optional, or to taste)

METHOD

1. No need for a juicer for this one, just blitz it all in a blender.

2. Add some water or apple juice if you want to make it a bit thinner or some crushed ice after a hot ride.

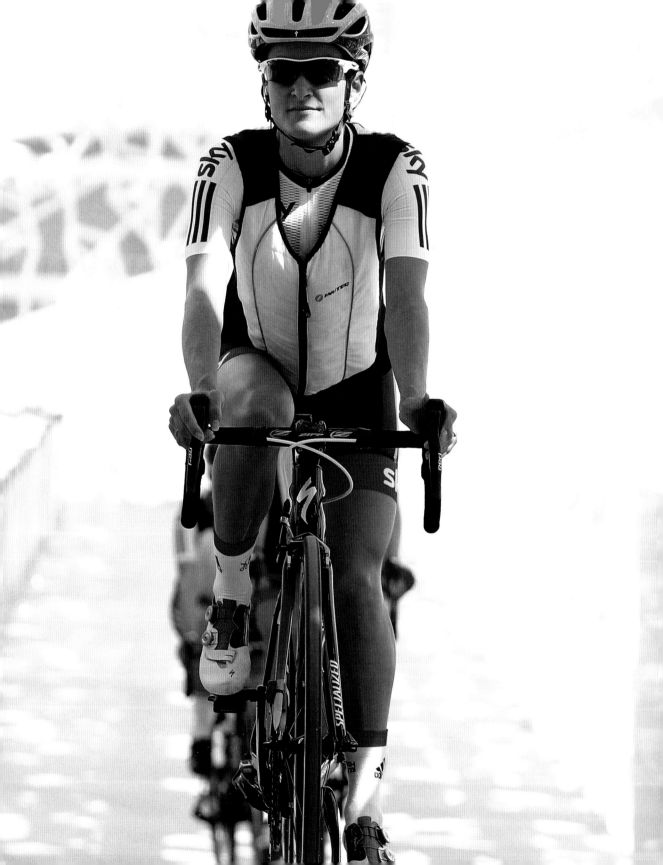

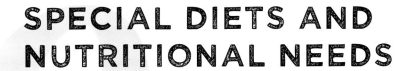

SPECIAL DIETS AND NUTRITIONAL NEEDS

Whether for health or, as is often the case for some vegetarians and vegans, ethical reasons, there are a number of special diets and nutritional needs that I have encountered and had to deal with during my career. Also, as with most top-level athletes, professional cyclists are always on the lookout for a new way to get that extra edge or a fast-track solution to lose a few pounds and this can mean latching onto the latest must-do nutritional fad that's currently passing through the peloton. More often than not, however, it's a case of guiding riders away from such spurious diets and getting them back onto the nutritional straight and narrow.

In this chapter, we look at vegetarian and vegan diets and how, with some thought, they can successfully support a cycling lifestyle. We also discuss two dietary interventions, going gluten- and lactose-free, which, although a health necessity for some people, have definitely become trendy, with reported performance benefits. Finally, we also look at some of the nutritional needs that are pertinent to female and junior cyclists.

VEGETARIANS AND VEGANS

I've actually worked with very few vegetarian and vegan cyclists, but that's not to say that you can't be one and be a highly successful cyclist. Becoming a vegetarian or a vegan is a personal choice and within those two blanket terms there's a whole spectrum of individuals. This ranges from people with ethical or moral objections to the exploitation of animals, who are completely vegan and won't eat animal by-products such as honey, to casual vegetarians who don't really enjoy the taste or texture of meat, but will occasionally have the odd piece of chicken or a bacon sandwich. Most of the riders I have worked with tended to fall into the latter camp and just didn't really enjoy eating meat, 2015

Lizzie Armitstead of Great Britain before the start of the Elite Women's Road Race during the UCI Road World Championships world road race champion Lizzie Armitstead being a notable example. Another top cyclist, David Zabriskie, an American pro, decided in 2010 that he wanted to follow a mainly plant-based diet, having salmon occasionally. As a nutritionist and a dietician, it's about looking at what the potential gaps in a vegetarian or vegan diet might be and how they can be filled. It's not that difficult, but in order to perform optimally, it does have to be considered. In this section I will provide an overview of some of the main considerations and recipes that are designed to help support vegetarian and vegan athletes.

Check that you're eating enough

Vegetarian and vegan diets tend to be high in fibre-rich foods which can fill you up quickly without delivering much calorific energy. This is great if you're trying to shed a kilo or two, but if you're in a heavy training block, it could leave you seriously under-fuelled. Keep a close eye on your body composition and how you're feeling on the bike, especially during higher-intensity workouts. If you think you're losing lean tissue mass or your power output on the bike is dropping, you could be under-fuelling yourself. If you're putting in big miles or hard efforts, you may have to resort to more refined and calorie-dense options such as white rice, pasta and potatoes.

COMPLETE PROTEINS

For vegetarians, your best sources of complete high-quality proteins are eggs and dairy, and if you're happy eating these there's no problem. For vegans, it's slightly trickier, as legumes (peas, beans and lentils), grains, nuts and seeds don't always individually contain a complete complement of essential amino acids. Without these amino acids, your body won't be able to synthesise the proteins to repair your muscles after hard training or maintain your lean muscle mass as effectively. Fortunately, by eating a wide variety of plant-based protein sources, you can cover all of your amino-acid bases. Brown rice and beans is a classic combination that will deliver a full complement of essential amino acids. There are also a number of plant-based protein sources, such as quinoa, buckwheat and soya, that are complete proteins.

A male cyclist will typically require 1.2–1.6 g/kg/day of protein, with female riders requiring 15 per cent less. This isn't a huge amount, but plant-based protein sources are far less protein-dense. For example, two turkey breasts will deliver about 40 g of protein, just under half the required amount for an 80 kg male rider, but to get the same from almonds, you'd have to eat over eight handfuls. This means that vegetarians and vegans may want to consider protein supplementation. For post-ride recovery, vegetarians will be able to use whey protein and there are a number of dedicated products that are soya based and suitable for vegans which deliver a complete protein in powder form from plant sources.

IRON

If you eat meat, the blood within it contains haemoglobin, which is an incredibly rich source of readily available iron. However, with foliate vegetables, such as spinach and broccoli, containing plenty of iron, there's no need for vegetarian and vegan cyclists to be deficient. Even using iron cookware can increase your iron intake as especially high acid foods encourage leaching of iron from the pan! However, the iron from plant-based sources may be harder for your body to absorb, but the process can be aided with organic acids. Vinegar in salad dressings, acid-containing tomatoes in the salad or a glass of orange juice with your meal are simple solutions. You should also look to avoid tea and coffee, which can both inhibit absorption. As we've already discussed in Chapters 1 and 9, iron deficiency can be an issue for all endurance athletes regardless of other dietary constraints. If you're regularly suffering from poor performance, fatigue or slow recovery, a blood test to confirm the deficiency and then supervised supplementation can be advisable.

B12

B12 and some of the other B vitamins are important for recovering from training, nerve function and for the creation of oxygen-carrying red blood cells. Vegetarians who eat dairy products have no worries, but vegans should consider supplementation. Fortunately, many foods, such as breakfast cereals or soy milk, are fortified with B12 and it's also present in most quality general multivitamins. Yeast extracts, such as Marmite, are good sources of general B vitamins and also tend to be fortified with B12. If you're in the camp that likes these spreads, they're a great addition to vegetarian and vegan diets.

CREATINE

As discussed in Chapter 9, creatine is important for sudden and explosive movements (see page 177). It is found in beef, pork and fish, but even for meat-eating riders, supplementation can definitely be a help during strength and hypertrophic (muscle building) phases of training. Studies have shown though that vegetarians can have lower levels of creatine in their muscles, so, if you're a track rider or a sprinter, you may want to consider supplementing it into your diet. Vegans need to be careful, however, as many supplemental creatine products are derived from shellfish, but there are other suitable ones available.

BETA-ALANINE

The supplement beta-alanine is an amino acid that acts as an acid buffer within the cell. It can be beneficial to multiple sprint performance, but as its usual source is from meat, vegetarians and vegans who are looking to improve this aspect of their riding may want to consider supplementing it into their diet.

ESSENTIAL FATTY ACIDS

One of the supplements that I have consistently recommended is a quality fish oil due to the omega-3 essential fatty acids they contain. Non-fish-eating vegetarians and vegans obviously can't take a fish- or krill-oil-based supplement, but with their diets commonly lacking in it, this is a gap that needs addressing. It's not as simple as just looking for foods which are high in omega-3 though, as it's the ratio with omega-6 which is important. You should therefore strive to increase your omega-3 intake while lowering that of omega-6. To lower omega-6 intake, avoid preparing foods with corn, sunflower, vegetable and sesame oils and instead opt for olive, avocado and peanut oils. To raise omega-3 intake, opt for flaxseeds, chia and hemp seeds. It does need to be milled or ground though as otherwise they will just pass straight through you. Milled flaxseed in particular is really good. You can also find omega-3 supplements specifically designed for vegetarians and vegans, which are often algae based.

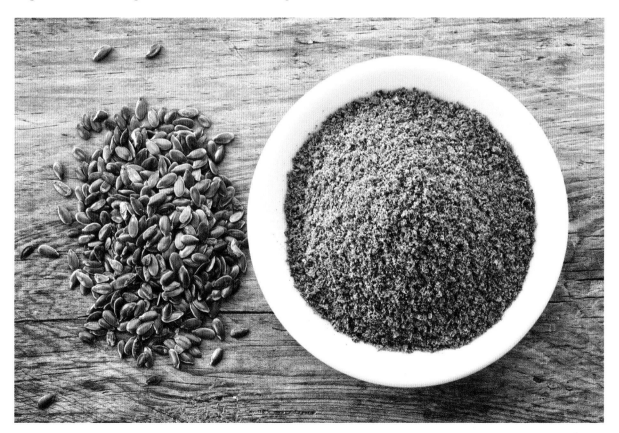

The peloton rides through the desert on stage four of the 2013 Tour of Qatar

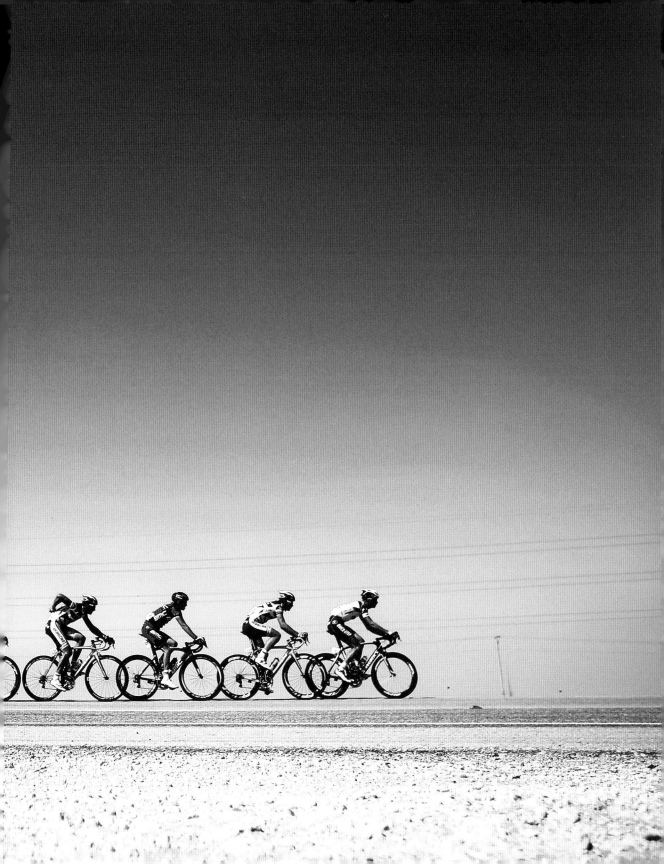

SLOW COOKER FIVE-BEAN CHILLI

This is one of my favourite recipes and at home we tend to have some version of this at least twice a week. It's great as the mix of beans gives a wide range of amino acids, especially when combined with rice. I will often add guacamole to go with it for some healthy fats and serve with tortilla wraps. I developed this recipe, as with most good recipes, through a specific need: my wife and youngest son are vegetarian. I tend to do the cooking, but, like most people, I can be short of time: so everything goes into the slow cooker and off you go!

Serves 6–8
Calories per serving:
   400 kcal
Carbohydrate per serving: 69 g
Fat per serving: 2.5 g
Protein per serving: 29 g

INGREDIENTS

200 g dried black-eyed peas
200 g dried butter beans
200 g dried haricot beans
   (navy beans)
200 g dried red kidney beans
200 g dried pinto beans
1 garlic clove, crushed
1 tbsp olive oil
2 medium onions, chopped
400 g can chopped tomatoes
2 tbsp tomato purée (tomato paste)
1 tbsp ground cumin
1 tbsp paprika
1 fresh chilli, finely chopped
   (2 tbsp ground chilli or more
   if you like it hot)
Salt and pepper, to taste
Approximately 2 l water

METHOD

1. Put the beans in the slow cooker and soak them overnight in about 1 litre of water.

2. In the morning, add the remaining ingredients, topping up with the rest of the water and switch onto a medium heat. The chilli should be ready in about eight hours. Serve with tortilla wraps, guacamole and lime wedges (optional).

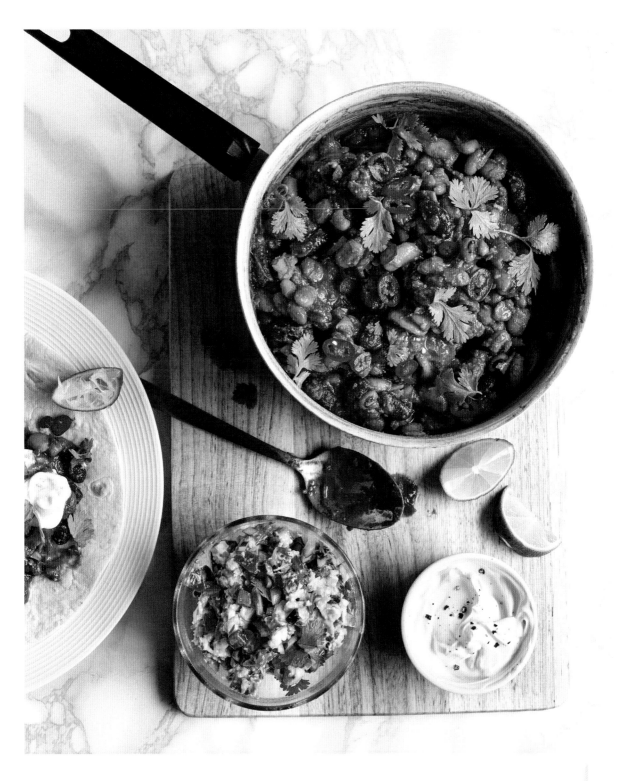

SOYA, CHIA AND FLAXSEED SMOOTHIE

This is a great vegan smoothie that can be used as a snack and is ideal as a recovery drink. This can form an ideal base to which you can add a few grams of creatine or a gram of beta-alanine. An alternative to the banana can be a handful of frozen berries.

Serves 1
Calories per serving: 253 kcal
Carbohydrate per serving: 18.4 g
Fat per serving: 12.5 g
Protein per serving: 12 g

INGREDIENTS

300 ml fortified unsweetened soya milk
1 small banana, peeled
1 tbsp flaxseeds
1 tbsp chia seeds

METHOD

1. This is really simple. Put all of the ingredients into a blender and blitz for about 30 seconds or until the drink has a smooth consistency.

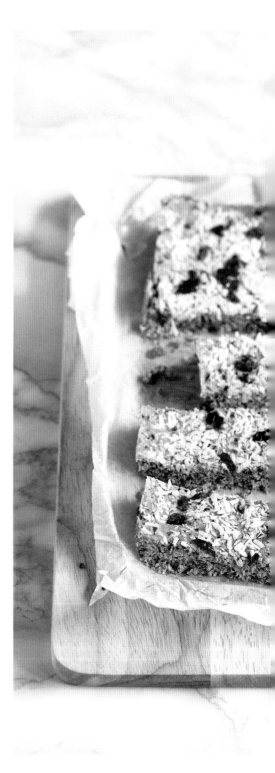

VEGAN PROTEIN BAR

These bars are extremely tasty and versatile. They can be used as a snack between meals, as recovery bars or wrap them in foil and take on the bike.

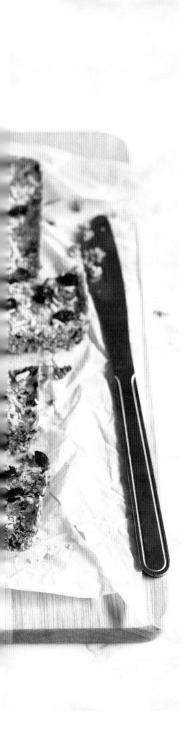

Servings 6 (6 bars)
Calories per serving:
   124 kcal
Carbohydrate per serving: 4.9 g
Fat per serving: 6.8 g
Protein per serving: 10 g

INGREDIENTS
60 g dried cranberries
60 g unflavored soya protein
60 g desiccated coconut
60 ml fortified unsweetened
   soya milk
1 tsp vanilla extract

METHOD

1. Place the cranberries in the bowl of a food processor and process until finely ground.

2. Add the coconut, soya protein and vanilla extract and process until the mixture is fine. The ideal texture should include small pieces of berries.

3. Add the soya milk and process until the mixture comes together.

4. Line a bar or loaf tin with greaseproof paper and press the mixture evenly into the tin using the back of a spoon.

5. Cover with clingfilm and refrigerate until it firms up (2-3 hours).

6. Cut into 6 equal-sized bars and keep in an airtight container.

GLUTEN-FREE

It wasn't so long ago that the staple diet of top-level cyclists was predominately wheat based. They'd eat huge amounts of pasta and bread, with high levels of carbohydrate intake seen as being crucial for endurance athletes. Even for non-athletes, wheat can easily dominate your diet. For many people, cereal at breakfast, a sandwich at lunchtime and then pasta in the evening can mean they're consuming wheat and gluten at every meal. Wheat is also present in many processed foods that we consume. For most people this isn't a problem, but, especially during periods of high-stress training loads, if gut health isn't optimal or because of certain medical conditions, it's not tolerated.

Gluten-free diets have become very popular in recent years, with riders and entire professional cycling teams very publicly praising the benefits of going gluten-free. Gluten is a protein composite that is found in wheat, barley, rye and a number of other grains. It gives dough its elastic properties, which helps it to rise, hold its shape during baking, and gives breads and cakes a light, springy texture. The rationale behind avoiding gluten is based on the fact that, unlike cows and some other mammals, we lack the enzymes in our saliva and stomach to fully break down and absorb gluten for nutritional use. This means that large blocks of undigested protein find their way into the small intestine, potentially slowing the absorption of other valuable nutrients, causing digestive stress and leading to feelings of fatigue and lethargy. Under the stressful conditions of heavy training or a stage race, such compromised digestion and energy levels are obvious problems that are worth avoiding, but for riders who don't suffer from any symptoms, the benefits of cutting gluten out of their diet are far from proven and much of the evidence is purely anecdotal. That said, a number of top riders are convinced of the benefits of cutting gluten during heavy racing and training blocks.

Medical reasons for avoiding gluten

There are three conditions which are genuine medical reasons for avoiding gluten and wheat.

Coeliac disease and dermatitis herpetiformis are well-recognised and serious autoimmune diseases, which, by eating gluten, trigger the body's immune system to turn on itself and attack the healthy tissue of the lower intestine. In particular, the finger-like projections known as villi are damaged. They become stunted and their ability to absorb nutrients is significantly reduced. Along with serious gastrointestinal distress and pain, this results in poor nutrient absorption, possible malnutrition and a constant feeling of tiredness. In some cases, individuals may also suffer from skin rashes. Some individuals can also have asymptomatic coeliac disease, where their only symptom is low energy or tiredness. A blood test will often reveal low iron levels due to poor absorption and this type of coeliac disease is far more common than we once suspected.

If you do suspect that you may be suffering from either of these conditions, it is essential to consult with your GP, rather than trying to remove gluten from your diet in an attempt to self-diagnose. The reason for this is that to obtain an accurate diagnosis of coeliac disease, gluten must have been present in the diet for a specified period before testing. It's important to obtain a diagnosis and begin treatment as, without it, there is a significantly increased risk of bowel cancer. People who suffer from noncoeliac gluten sensitivity and intolerance can display many of the symptoms of coeliac disease, such as headaches, bloating, fatigue and diarrhoea, but do not have damage to their intestinal lining.

Wheat allergies are more common in children and often resolve as they become older, but they can also be present in adults. Allergies are where the body recognises a protein within a food as being alien and has an acute immune response to it. At the most extreme of the spectrum, this reaction can result in life-threatening anaphylactic shock, with peanut allergies being especially dangerous. However, wheat allergies tend to be less severe, with the symptoms being similar to the previously described conditions, but can also include asthma-like symptoms, eczema and other skin irritations.

One high-profile athlete who suffered from undiagnosed coeliac disease for twelve years was British track sprinter Craig MacLean. Having won silver at the Sydney Olympics in 2000, he was plagued by extreme exhaustion, anaemia and muscle cramps in his build-up to the 2008 Beijing Olympics. Just before the Games, he lost his place on Team GB. He continued training, accepting the cycles of pain and extreme exhaustion, and, still undiagnosed, won gold in the men's sprint with Anthony Kappes at the London 2012 Paralympics. It was one year after that he was finally diagnosed with coeliac disease. There's no doubt the condition compromised his career as a cyclist and what he did manage to achieve is a massive testament to his talent and dedication.

Is it worth trying a gluten-free diet?

If you don't suffer from any of the conditions described above, it's debatable whether there's anything to gain from going gluten-free. However, if you're training or racing hard and are suffering from gastrointestinal discomfort, it can be worth reducing the amount of gluten in your diet. However, you should also work through all of the other steps for maintaining optimal gut health discussed in Chapter 2. Also, if you're following the gut rehab plan (see pages 32–34) after a gastrointestinal disturbance or a course of antibiotics, gluten should be cut from the diet. Remember though, there have been riders that have come to teams who I've been working with and who initially claimed to be gluten intolerant, but, after working on their gut health, would happily tuck into a baguette, having been 'cured'.

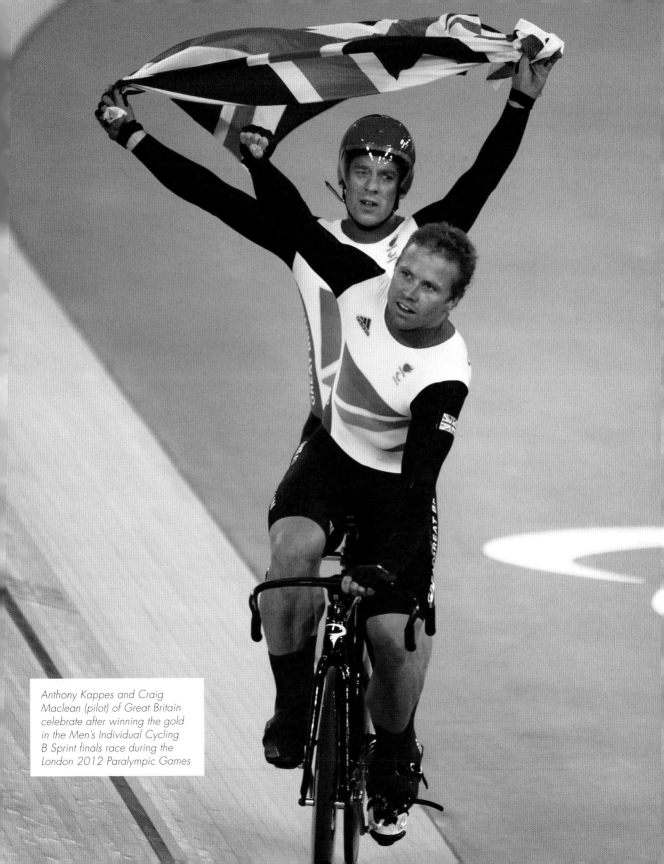

Anthony Kappes and Craig Maclean (pilot) of Great Britain celebrate after winning the gold in the Men's Individual Cycling B Sprint finals race during the London 2012 Paralympic Games

Gluten-free eating

If you choose to avoid wheat and gluten, you're also cutting out a great source of fibre. Fibre is not only essential for healthy bowel function, but is also vital as a prebiotic for good bacteria in the gut, which uses it for energy. Make sure you're replacing this fibre with fruit and vegetables. If your gut is sensitive, for whatever reason, you can get this fibre in a gut-friendly way by using vegetable juices. Bread and pasta are a convenient source of carbohydrates, but they're easy to replace with starchy root vegetables, such as potatoes, sweet potatoes and yams. The breakfast option I recommend to all riders is porridge. It has previously been advised that oats should be avoided if you require a gluten-free diet due to the high probability of contamination in the factory by gluten-containing grains, however, there are now oats available that are guaranteed and labelled as gluten-free. You can also use a number of other grains, such as quinoa, buckwheat and millet. For some people who are not coeliac or gluten intolerant, but might just be suffering from wheat overload in their diet, there are a number of other grains you can try. Rye and spelt are good examples and, although containing gluten, can be good if you're just wanting to reduce your intake of wheat itself.

On the bike, going gluten-free isn't a problem. You can use the rice cakes from Chapter 6 (see pages 112–113) and there are many gluten-free bars commercially available now. Most gels use maltodextrin and glucose syrup as energy sources and, although both can be derived from wheat and other grains, the manufacturing process removes the gluten. Many energy drink mixes do contain gluten though as they include ingredients such as waxy starches and you should carefully check the ingredients before using. An option would be to mix your own energy drinks using the recipes in Chapter 3 (see pages 56–57).

DAIRY-FREE

Lactose is the sugar found in milk and a lactose intolerance is where people don't produce the enzyme lactase which breaks down this sugar. For these people, if exposed to lactose, they'll suffer from gastrointestinal issues, such as bloating and diarrhoea. The only treatment is to totally avoid foods containing lactose or to take lactase supplements. There are, however, degrees of intolerance and sensitivity and whether you suffer a reaction will depend on the amount of lactose you consume. For example, you may not be able to tolerate drinking a pint of milk, but are fine with yoghurt or some cheese. The main reason for this is that some of the lactose is already broken down by the bacteria in the yoghurt or cheese cultures. You can also be intolerant or sensitive to the milk proteins, giving rise to similar symptoms to above.

A number of athletes find when training or racing hard that a high level of dairy in their diet can lead to an increase in phlegm production. For this reason, a number of riders I've worked with will cut down on dairy during key races and training camps. Also, if you're following the gut rehab plan (see page 32–34), you should cut out dairy as it can be stressful to an already compromised digestive system.

The main issue with cutting dairy from your diet is ensuring that you replace the calcium and protein that it provides. Some people who struggle with dairy products find that they are absolutely fine with protein products containing whey protein. This is because the whey protein is often hydrolysed (broken down with a chemical reaction involving water) during the manufacturing process, so it is easier to digest, or the whey is isolated so there aren't any of the other components in the milk present which can be the irritants. If you can't tolerate these products, you'll need to ensure you're getting adequate protein from another source, and there are a number of plant-based products available that you could try. For calcium, the best non-dairy sources are leafy greens, seafood and legumes. You'll also find that many foods, such as bread, breakfast cereals and non-dairy milk alternatives, are fortified with calcium.

The table on page 206 is a quick reference guide to all of the recipes in the book as to their suitability for vegetarians, vegans and those following gluten- or lactose-free diets.

Recipe	Chapter	Vegetarian	Vegan	Gluten free	Lactose free
Homemade Sports Drinks 1 and 2	3	✓	✓	✓	✓
Turkey Breast Steak with Homemade Sweet Potato Wedges and Wilted Spinach	4			✓	✓
Pistachio Pâté with Homemade Sweet Potato Wedges and Wilted Spinach	4	✓	✓	✓	✓
Chicken Breast in a Simple Tomato Sauce on a Bed of Rice and Quinoa	4			✓	✓
Perfect Porridge	5	✓	✓*	✓**	✓*
Omelette	5	✓		✓	✓
Quinoa and Coconut Milk Porridge	5	✓	✓	✓	✓
Chocolate, Seed, Nut and Berry Porridge Topping	5	✓	✓	✓	✓
Rice Cakes	6	✓		✓	
Homemade Energy Balls	6	✓	✓	✓**	✓
Traditional Panini	6	✓			
DIY Recovery Drink	7	✓		✓	
Slow Cooker Recovery Stew	7			✓	✓
Recovery-boosting Mackerel and Tomato Salad	7	✓***		✓	✓
Turkey Burgers	8			✓	✓
Caprese Salad	8	✓		✓	
Very Berry Protein Fluff	8	✓			
Turkey Power Soup	9			✓	✓
Beetroot Juice	9	✓	✓	✓	✓
Super-green Smoothie	9	✓		✓	
Slow Cooker Five Bean Chilli	10	✓	✓	✓	✓
Soya, Chia and Flaxseed Smoothie	10	✓	✓	✓	✓
Vegan Protein Bar	10	✓	✓	✓	✓

* If made with water
** Check oats are gluten free certified
*** Suitable for pescatarians

FEMALE RIDERS

At both a recreational and competitive level, women's cycling is on the rise. This is great to see and, with my mother and her sisters being the main reason I got into cycling, personally gratifying. Although the basic principles of nutrition are the same, I've found that female cyclists do have some specific requirements. It's not just about scaling down a bit what we do with men.

A fairly high proportion of women of reproductive age may suffer from heavy menstrual bleeding. This can lead to low iron levels which, in combination with heavy training and racing that also reduces iron levels, can cause anaemia and the associated symptoms of fatigue, poor recovery and reduced performance. You should consult a medical professional to have a blood test to confirm low iron levels before considering supplementation.

All top-level cyclists tend to be weight conscious, but I've often found female riders to be even more so. It's definitely worth remembering that when you want to train hard, it isn't the time to try and lose weight. I've often found that female riders will restrict their food intake on the bike and will then find themselves playing catch-up with their energy balance and compromising their training. You have to provide the fuel for your training. If you fuel well on the bike, you'll be able to ride harder and for longer than if you're attempting to train on a restrictive diet.

For competitive female cyclists, race volume and therefore training volume will typically be lower than for men. However, the intensity of women's racing is as high and so the muscle damage will be significant. This means that you should pay particular attention to the recovery guidelines described in Chapter 7. Make sure you're eating enough high-quality protein, which, for female riders, is about 1–1.4 g/kg of bodyweight/day. Also ensure that you're getting enough calcium as this is very important for bone health. Don't be fearful of fat. Healthy fats from nuts and seeds, avocados, oily fish or omega-3 supplements are essential for general health, performance and hormone production within your body.

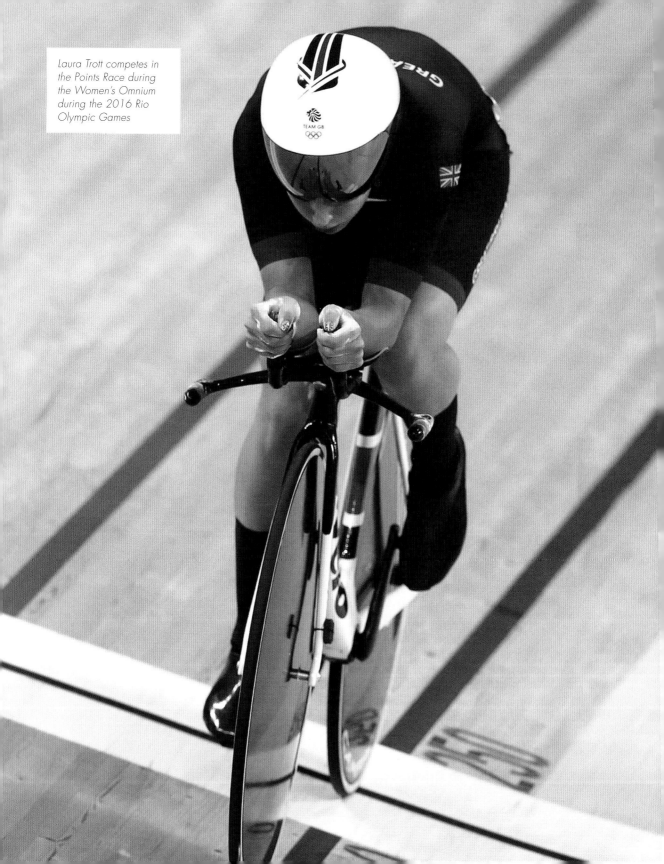

PRO STORY: GREAT BRITAIN'S CYCLING HEROINES

Britain has a rich history of successful women cyclists. This goes right back to Beryl Burton, who used to compete against my mother in the 1950s and dominated women's cycling racing in the UK – she even set a 12-hour time trial record which wasn't bettered by anyone, male or female, for two years. In recent years we have had riders such as Nicole Cook, Victoria Pendleton and the current stars include Dame Sarah Storey, Joanna Rowsell Shand, Becky James and Laura Trott.

There are considerable differences in both the training regimes and nutritional needs across the cycling disciplines. Track sprinters have to spend a lot of time in the gym, lifting heavy weights to build strength and explosive power. Their efforts on the track are very short, intense and have long rest periods to allow full recovery. The priority for them is providing the protein and calories to support muscle growth and repair. Female athletes on the whole tend to find it more difficult than their male counterparts to gain muscle mass and, if they do, those gains are easily lost. Much of this is down to a difference in hormonal make up, especially the relative levels of testosterone in men and women. However, by ensuring that their protein intake is optimal and providing the correct training stimuli, female riders can achieve strength and muscle gains. Female riders shouldn't shy away from strength training because of the fear of 'bulking up' too much. I can assure you that even when top female track sprinters are doing everything they can to gain muscle, it's always an uphill battle.

For injury prevention, increased metabolic rate, bone health and performance on the bike, almost all female riders could benefit from some time in the gym. Track endurance riders, such as Joanna Rowsell Shand and Laura Trott, are spending more time in the gym building strength and power. However, they still put in massive road miles and their track sessions are a brutal combination of intensity, duration and short recoveries. They require more carbohydrates around their training sessions than their sprinter team-mates, but, for recovery and to build and maintain muscle mass, they also need a good amount of quality protein.

JUNIOR RIDERS

It's definitely worth highlighting the nutritional needs of young riders who are still developing. The first consideration is that these young riders are also growing and developing, which uses up huge amounts of energy. It's essential that they're getting the calories they require. Well-meaning parents may provide their children with a super-healthy diet which is low in sugar and fat, but if your child is very active, the priority is giving them the calories they need. If a young rider is training hard, you can afford to be a bit more relaxed, and some of the sugary foods that are perceived as being unhealthy can ensure they're getting the energy they need. Make sure they're also getting a good amount of quality protein and plenty of bright fruit and vegetables for the 'glow nutrients'. Calcium, from dairy or foliate vegetables, is also very important.

Teenagers will go through growth spurts and periods of maturation when they just want to sleep the whole time and you'll typically see the quality of training they're able to do drop off. This is because the body is having to devote a huge amount of energy to growth, so it's essential that this energy is provided in their diet.

Finally, on the bike, younger riders' metabolisms are less efficient and so they have to fuel more regularly. They burn a far higher percentage of carbohydrate than a mature rider and can go from riding strongly one moment to an abrupt halt 50 metres down the road. A friend of mine has a 15-year-old son who would ride really well for 90 minutes, but then blow up. I found that he just wasn't eating enough on the bike. This problem is compounded by the fact that younger riders are very easily distracted and will simply forget to eat. If you are the parent or coach of a budding Sir Bradley Wiggins or Lizzie Armitstead, make sure they are eating and drinking regularly right from the start of their ride. Explain why it's important to them – a car and fuel analogy always works well. Remind them to eat if you're with them or, if not, put an 'Eat!' note on their stem. I have to do this with some professional riders so they remember to eat, so you can tell young riders that!

KNOWLEDGE TO TAKE AWAY

- **Be suspicious of fads** *Don't be fooled by the latest must-do miracle diet for weight loss or performance gains. I can almost guarantee it won't live up to the hype and won't deliver the results it promises.*

- **Vegetarians and vegans can be great athletes** *There's no reason why you can't be a successful competitive cyclist following a vegetarian or vegan diet. You just need to take care to fill in some of the potential nutritional gaps that such diets can cause.*

- **Going gluten- or dairy-free isn't a magic bullet** *Unless you have a diagnosed medical condition, such as coeliac disease or lactose intolerance, the benefits of cutting out gluten and dairy are far from proven. However, under extreme training stress, following a gastrointestinal disturbance or if you've overdone foods containing wheat or dairy, cutting down or cutting out for a period of time can be beneficial.*

- **Female riders have different needs** *The general nutritional guidelines outlined in this book apply equally to female riders as to their male counterparts. However, there are a few areas that require more attention or a slightly different approach.*

- **Make sure junior riders get enough fuel** *Young riders require a lot of calories to fuel their training and growth, both on and off the bike. Take steps to ensure they remember to fuel little, often and early on their rides, and although a healthy diet is important, don't worry too much about the odd sweet or sugary drink.*

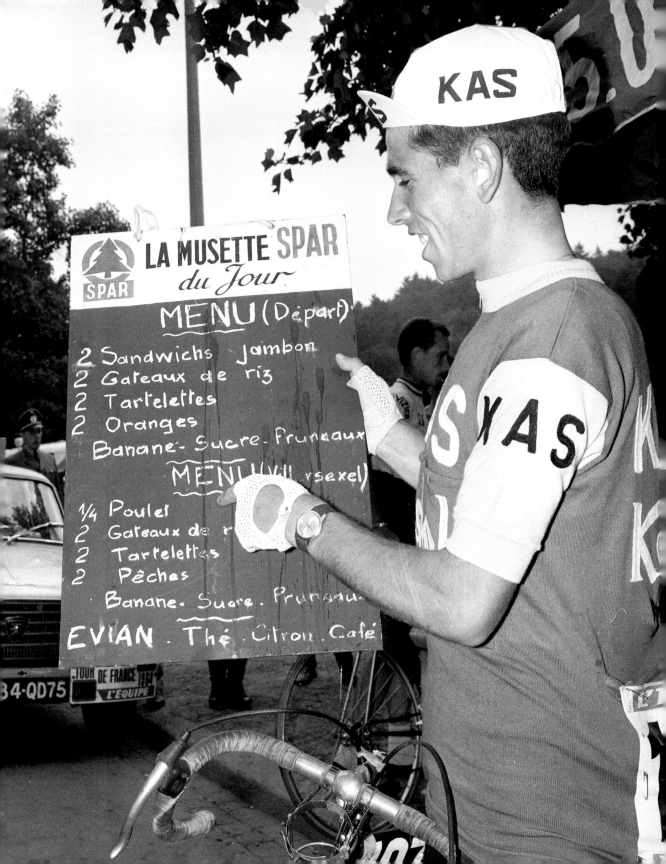

NUTRITIONAL TIMELINES

Having been through in detail how you can optimise your nutrition for both cycling performance and health, this chapter provides a quick reference guide to when and what to eat for a number of cycling scenarios. It's important to remember though that all riders are individual and, as with all aspects of sports science and performance, need to be treated as such. Follow the advice given in this chapter and throughout the book, but experiment in training and at less important events to tweak it to your specific needs and physiology.

If you're struggling to get your cycling nutrition right, go back to basics. Take steps to improve your gut health, following the recommendations in Chapter 2 (see pages 25–39). Try a number of alternatives from the recipes in the book for fuelling before, during and after rides. Allow a bit more time between your pre-ride meal and actually riding. Experiment with the frequency and amount of food you take on while riding. Use a heart rate monitor or power meter to monitor your riding intensity and ensure you're not pushing too hard for your current fitness level.

The exact times of your events or rides may differ to those given here but you can easily shift the timeline to fit your needs. You'll notice that many of the routines are very similar and this is because the basic principles of sound nutrition are applicable across cycling disciplines.

SPORTIVE OR LONG TRAINING RIDE: 9 A.M. START

For a sportive, where you may be looking to ride a certain time or get round quicker than your mates, you need to be a bit more disciplined about your nutrition, especially if there are long climbs, than on a training ride. This starts the day before so, review the

Joaquim Galera, Spanish racing cyclist, presenting the menu of a stage of the 1964 Tour de France

information in Chapter 4, and if you're having to travel to the event or stay over, make sure your nutrition is at the top of your logistical priorities.

6 a.m.: Don't forget to set your alarm! You need three to four hours between your breakfast and starting your event. Aim to consume 1 g of carbohydrate per kg of bodyweight. An ideal breakfast would be a bowl of porridge with seed and berry topping and a banana chopped into it. Add an omelette or some yoghurt for protein. Keep sipping on a sports drink to top up your carbohydrates or plain water if you feel you've had enough, and if you like a coffee, have a couple of espressos as they can give you a bit of a boost.

6.30-8.30 a.m.: Keep sipping on your sports drink. You should try to consume about 500 ml per hour in the lead-up to your start. Have a couple of light snacks, about one each hour. Opt for an energy bar, rice cakes or a banana.

8.30-9.00 a.m.: Get to the start area with plenty of time to spare and have a final visit to the bathroom. Don't set off too hard. You've practised your pacing in training, so stick to your tried-and-tested plan.

9.10 a.m.: First sip from your water bottle. Continue taking one every 10–15 minutes throughout the ride.

9.20-9.45 a.m.: First feed of the ride. Exact frequency will depend on riding intensity and personal preference. You should be aiming to consume 20–30 g of carbohydrates every 30–45 minutes. All of the on-the-bike recipes in Chapter 6 deliver close to this figure. Keep feeding in this way throughout the ride.

Five minutes before a big climb: Especially on continental sportives with really long climbs, a gel just before hitting the early ramps can give you an instant boost and fuel the higher-intensity effort. Also, try to eat something as you crest the climb as the lower-intensity effort needed as you descend offers a great chance for easier digestion.

Feed stations: If you're looking to perform optimally, my advice is to be nutritionally self-sufficient and just use the feed stations to re-fill your bottles. If you do decide to take some food from the feed station, try to ensure it's something you've used on a ride before and incorporate it into your overall fuelling strategy. Overeating can be as bad as under-eating. If your goal is a more leisurely day out, enjoy the cakes!

Final hour: Keep disciplined and carry on eating and drinking. Don't skip a feed because you only think there's a few kilometres to go. A caffeinated gel can give you an extra final boost. If you start to bonk, don't think that a gel won't have time to work, as the sweetness in your mouth alone will give you an instant lift.

Finish: Protein is your priority. Consume a 20 g serving of whey protein or similar in 500 ml of water as soon after finishing as possible.

EVENING CRIT OR 10-MILE TIME TRIAL: 7 P.M. START

Often held mid-week, meaning you may have a working day beforehand, and fairly high intensity, these 20-minute to one-hour type events can be tricky to fuel for. You don't want to eat too much too close to the race and risk feeling bloated or nauseous, but equally you don't want to underperform because you've consumed too little.

1 p.m.: Although your race is still six hours away, what you have for lunch can have a significant effect on how you perform. An ideal lunch would be a chicken or tuna salad followed by a pot of natural yoghurt and then make sure you're constantly sipping water and staying hydrated throughout the rest of the day.

3 p.m.: A mid-afternoon snack is vital to avoid a late afternoon energy crash that could leave you weak for your race. Make sure you have some healthy snacks to hand, such as nuts, seeds, an apple, pear, bowl of sugar-free cereal or muesli, yoghurt, rice cake or an energy bar.

5 p.m.: This is your absolute latest window for solid food. Both a 10-mile time trial and a crit are high-intensity events and you don't want to risk the effort involved causing you to feel, or even be, sick. An energy bar or a bowl of cereal are good choices and again, especially if it's warm, drinking little and often is essential.

6.30 p.m.: You'll be at the race HQ and, if you haven't ridden to the event, will have either started or just be starting your warm-up. Keep drinking and, in the hour leading up to the race, aim to consume 500–750 ml of fluid.

6.45 p.m.: Fifteen minutes before the race start you should be coming to the end of your warm-up, so take an energy gel with the remaining liquid in your bottle. Some riders like to use a caffeinated gel at this stage, but be aware that it could affect the quality of your sleep afterwards. This should leave you with five to 10 minutes before the start, plenty of time for a final toilet stop and then to make your way to the line.

7 p.m. (the race): For a 10-mile time trial, there should be no need to eat or drink for the entirety of the event. Coming out of your aero tuck to reach for a bottle or gel will lose time, break your rhythm and reduce focus. For a typical 45- to 60-minute circuit race, your pre-race nutrition and hydration should be adequate. If it's hot, a

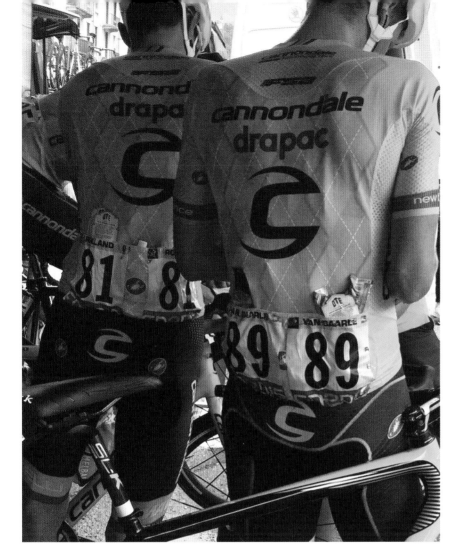

500 ml bottle of sports drink is good idea. Take a decent gulp towards the crescendo of the race for the sugar-in-your-mouth boost.

8 p.m. *(post-race)*: Have a recovery drink that delivers about 20 g of protein and, if you won't eating soon after the event, 20–30 g of carbohydrate. Remember to factor this into your meal when you do get home though so you don't overeat. You can have this as you do your cool-down, as you ride home or back at the car. Don't worry too much about carbohydrates as you won't have depleted your stores and can easily top them up once you get home.

8.30 p.m. - bedtime: Once home, you probably won't want to eat a full meal this late and it could interfere with your sleep. A light snack such as some cereal or beans on toast would be ideal. When I suggest cereal, I'm referring to a low-sugar choice, such as a quality muesli.

Track league

Another event that falls into this time slot is an evening track league. With multiple short but very intense events, along with warming up and cooling down on rollers, and typically lasting for two hours or more, fuelling has to be slightly different. Follow the guidelines above for the afternoon and build-up, then make these small tweaks.

Fluid and salt loss can be a real issue in the 25 °C (77° F) plus temperature of an indoor velodrome, so you should be sipping on a sports drink with electrolytes throughout the meeting. Don't be surprised if you get through 1.5–2 l. With the extremely high-intensity nature of the racing, you'll probably also require some additional fuel. Three or four gels over the course of the evening's racing wouldn't be excessive. Take one during your first warm-up as described above and then space the others across evening. Take them during the cool-downs following races. If you take them before, they can repeat on you during the abrupt top-end sprint efforts associated with track racing. The muscle load and damage from track racing is high, so protein is definitely your recovery priority. Although the race meeting will have lasted two hours, the actual time spent riding hard is fairly short. You should still only need a light snack when you get home.

EARLY-MORNING TIME TRIAL: 8 A.M. START

Many time trials have very early start times. This isn't just a tradition that harks back to the days when the sport was frowned upon by the authorities and conducted in secret, but is due to the lower early-morning traffic volume.

5 a.m.: If you want to have a full breakfast, this is the time that you'll have to be eating it at. At that time in the morning, eating can be hard, so keep it light and digestible. Some muesli with yoghurt, a small bowl of porridge, poached eggs on toast or even a banana and oat smoothie can all work well. Don't forget though, as long as you've eaten well the day before, your glycogen reserves will already be well stocked up.

A full breakfast is probably necessary for any event longer than 80 kilometres, but for shorter ones my recommendation is to set your alarm an hour or so later and opt for rice pudding. Try it at a couple of less important events or in training; many riders can even tolerate it without any adverse effects as close to an hour before a hard race effort. Have a coffee if you normally do, and as you travel to the HQ and throughout the morning, sip on a bottle of sports drink or plain water, depending on your requirements.

7 a.m.: Arriving at the Race HQ, sign on, pick up your race number, find out your start time, and working back from your start time, begin your warm-up so that you finish it 15 minutes before your allocated start time.

7.45-7.55 a.m.: Towards the end of your warm-up take a gel. Some riders like to use a caffeinated one but make sure you've tried this in training. Go to the bathroom if you need to, make your way to the start and keep sipping on your bottle.

8 a.m. (the race): For a 25-mile (40-kilometre) time trial, you can probably ride it without taking on any extra fuel or fluids. However, for the boost it'll give you for the tough final quarter, I'd recommend taking a gel at about the halfway mark. Don't worry if your skin suit hasn't got pockets, just stash it up your leg. For a 50-mile (80-kilometre) event, you'd probably want to break it into thirds and have a gel at one-third and two-thirds of the distance. For longer events, which will be ridden at a lower intensity, your fuelling will be more akin to a sportive and you should be looking to take in 20–30 g of carbohydrates every 30–45 minutes. You should also consider using slower-burn solid food, such as rice cakes and energy bars, rather than just gels for longer events.

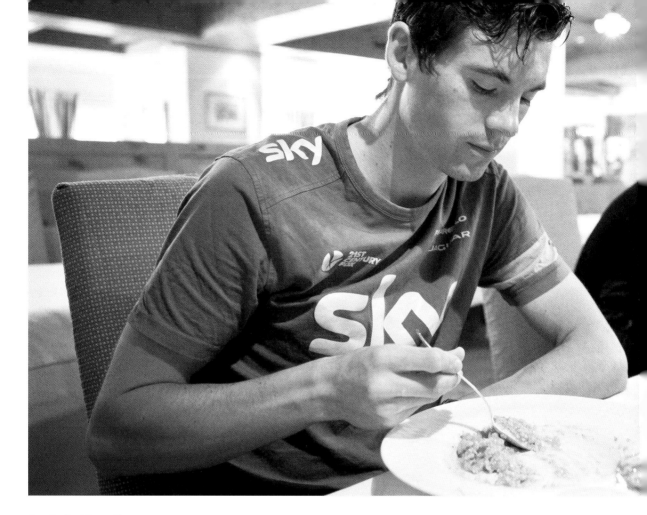

Ben Swift of Team Sky eats breakfast during the 2014 Giro d'Italia

Post-ride: You'll finish a 25- or a 50-mile (40- or 80-kilometre) time trial well before lunchtime. Have a protein drink as you cool down and this should see you though to lunchtime when something like the Mackerel Salad from Chapter 7 would be ideal (see pages 138–139). If lunch is likely to be more than two to three hours away, pack a sandwich or a salad in a cool-box. Even though your ride was hard, it won't have been that long, so there's no need to eat excessive amounts. For longer events, if you've fuelled well on the bike, a protein drink is still your priority on finishing. Again, if your next proper meal is more than two to three hours away, plan ahead, pack a snack and don't end up relying on roadside service stations.

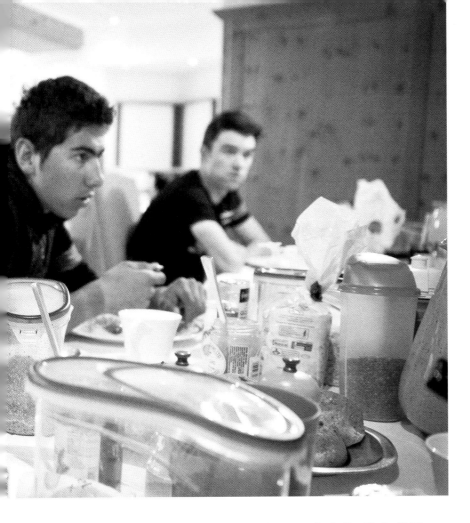

MID-MORNING CYCLOCROSS RACE: 10 A.M. START

With cold winter conditions and technical high-intensity racing, cyclocross is demanding on riders, bikes and their supporters.

7 a.m.: For a cyclocross race starting at 10 a.m., a 7 a.m. breakfast will allow you three hours to fully digest it. You don't need to eat a huge amount, but equally, you don't want to be feeling weak or hungry on the start line. Remember, it's likely to be cold so choosing a hot option can give you a warming boost and, as ever, porridge is ideal. Have some coffee if it's normally part of your breakfast and sip on fluids throughout the morning.

8-9 a.m.: During your journey to the race, keep sipping on your water bottle. Arrive at the Race HQ, sign on, pick up your race number, double-check your race start time and get your warm-up kit on. You might want a light snack, such as an energy bar, banana or rice cake, during this period, especially if your start time is later.

9.20-9.45 a.m.: Ride your warm-up on the course if possible to become familiar with it and keep a bottle in your jersey or jacket pocket to take occasional sips from between harder efforts. An insulated bottle containing green tea with sugar or honey can give you a welcome bit of extra warmth. Aim to finish your warm-up 15–20 minutes before the start of the race. You might want to take an energy gel at this point and some riders like to use a caffeinated one. This will leave you time to strip down to your race kit, make any last-minute adjustments to tyre pressure based on your warm-up laps and have a final bathroom stop before heading to the start.

10 a.m. (the race): With a cyclocross race lasting 30–60 minutes there's no need to take on any food or drink, and with the full-on and technical nature of the racing, you won't have any real chance to either.

Post-ride: Once you've finished, dried yourself with a towel and got some clean and dry clothes on, have a protein shake. My recommendation for cyclocross is to choose chocolate flavor; make it up with hot water beforehand and have it warm and ready in a thermos for when you've finished. This protein drink is all you really need until lunchtime, but again, if your lunch is likely to be delayed by more than two to three hours, have a snack to eat in the car. If you're organized, you'll have my recovery stew from Chapter 7 (see pages 136–137) bubbling in your slow cooker at home waiting for you.

WORKING DAY WITH COMMUTES

For many amateur riders, their commute to and from work is where they get the bulk of their miles in.

Ride in and breakfast

It's not realistic on a working day to allow two to three hours of digestion after your breakfast before heading off for your ride to work. My recommendation is to get up, have a cup of black tea or coffee, get on your bike and use your morning commute as a metabolic carbohydrate-fasted ride. See Chapter 6 for full details and remember you can have a bottle of protein drink as you ride and still get the fat oxidation and efficiency benefits of this type of training.

Once you get to work, porridge again provides an ideal start to your day. You can use a microwave or use a porridge pot that you just add boiling water to.

11 a.m.: It's been a couple of hours since breakfast and hunger can strike. It is really important to keep your blood sugar levels up, as this will keep your concentration and motivation levels high through the working day and more importantly for the next ride. As we move through the day a lot of people do not maintain a good blood sugar level, one of the mistakes is that they often go too long before they eat. A mid-morning snack will maintain blood sugar and energy levels. This snack can be very simple, such as a banana and natural yoghurt, or a handful of nuts and seeds with an apple.

1 p.m.: You're far more likely to eat well if you bring your own lunch in with you and avoid the work canteen or the dash to the sandwich bar. I'm a big fan of making an extra portion of whatever you have for dinner and taking that in for lunch the next day. Another option is to do some bulk cooking at the weekend and freeze portions for your lunches the next week. Sir Bradley Wiggins' inflight choice of Chicken Breast in a Simple Tomato

Sauce on a Bed of Rice and Quinoa from Chapter 4 is ideal, as are the Turkey Power Soup (page 185) and the Slow Cooker Recovery Stew recipes (see pages 136–137).

3 p.m.: If you're planning on riding home and either upping the intensity or adding some extra miles, a mid-afternoon snack is essential. Even if not, you should have something to avoid an energy crash, which can lead to you snacking on junk. Ideally you should aim to eat it two hours before you're planning to ride. It needs to be something that is easy on the stomach and can be digested easily. This could be a banana and some yoghurt, cereal or, if you had that in the morning, then treat yourself to a small piece of flapjack. If you're not riding home, still have a snack, but just have some orchard fruit and maybe some nuts or seeds.

5 p.m.: If your commute home is under 90 minutes, you shouldn't need any extra fuel, but if you're going longer than this, go straight into the usual routine of a sip from your bottle every 10–15 minutes to keep hydrated and 20–30 g of carbohydrate every 30–45 minutes for fuelling.

Back at home: If your ride has been more than 90 minutes and/or has included some hard interval type efforts, you should have a protein drink when you get in. You should then aim to have your dinner within 2–3 hours. Think about the riding you'll be doing the next day and use that to dictate the amount of carbohydrates you consume but there's no need to eat excessive amounts, 50 g is plenty enough for a typical weekday evening meal. This could be a medium sized sweet potato, two and a half slices of wholemeal bread or 85 g of cooked basmati rice. A piece of chicken, fish or steak weighing about 200 g is going to provide ample protein or, if you're vegetarian or vegan, look at Chapter 10 for suitable alternatives. Don't forget vegetables or salad for those 'glow nutrients' and to make an extra portion for lunch the next day.

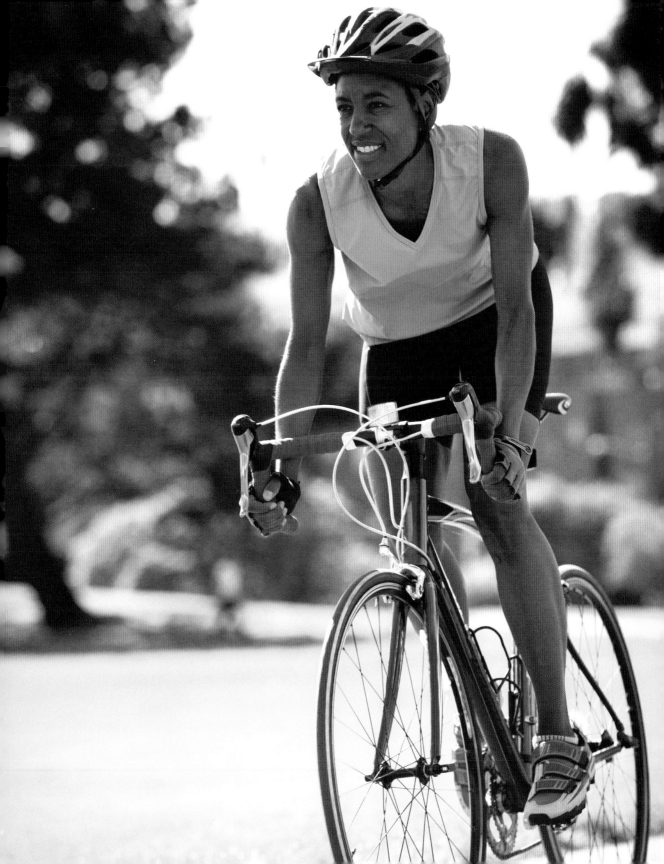

PRO STORY: THE GRAND TOUR TIME TRIAL

My first year with Team Sky was a real eye-opener into how seriously the team took logistics and taking the time to ensure that every detail was examined with an end goal of improved performance. At the 2010 Giro d'Italia, which began with an 8.4 km prologue time trial, one of my main tasks was optimising the riders' pre-race meal. Time trials and prologues are especially demanding as all the riders are setting off at different times and, as the effort is so intense, pre-race fuelling has to be spot-on. Too late or too indigestible and the rider will feel bloated and nauseous; too early or too light and the rider will feel weak and unpowered.

The solution is to work back from each rider's start time and to provide a flexible meal option that they can eat at the optimum time for their ride. So, if a rider is off at 4 p.m., their pre-race meal would be between 12 p.m. and 1 p.m. and their breakfast would be at 9 a.m. This means that their pre-race meal had to be given to them on the team bus. I'd get the chef to cook extra omelettes in the morning and then we'd pack them up and put them in the fridge on the bus. I'd have a rice cooker on the bus and so the riders would be able to have an ideal and easily digestible pre-race meal of rice omelettes at exactly the time they needed it.

They would then be able to chill out on the team bus, keep sipping on fluids and then get onto their turbo for their warm-up, maybe with a gel, in exactly the same way as described for a club TT described above. That was the first Grand Tour that Team Sky had ridden and it got off to a great start with Sir Bradley Wiggins winning that opening time trial. Rice and omelette has now become one of the staple pre-race meals across all cycling disciplines and levels of competition.

The main lesson that you can learn from this is that forward preparation and good logistics are essential for optimum performance. If you've put in hours of training for a big event, you don't want to blow it with a bad stomach. Invest in a cool box, cook yourself an omelette and some rice or, if you're travelling on the day before an event, use a recipe such as chicken, tomato sauce, rice and quinoa from Chapter 4. You didn't compromise on your training, so don't compromise on your nutritional preparation. Be organized and leave nothing to chance.

KNOWLEDGE TO TAKE AWAY

- **Plan** Whether it's a key training session, your local club 10-mile time trial, a sportive or a National Championships, plan your nutrition and create your own timeline.

- **Adapt** Use training and less important events to test and refine your timeline. Recreate the time of day you'll be competing at, and having used the advice in this book to create your template, fine-tune it to your individual needs. Remember, we're all different, so what might work perfectly for your main rival or Laura Trott might need adjusting for you.

- **Prepare** Once you've worked out a timeline that works for you and your event, do everything you can to stick to it. Whether that's pre-preparing some meals or checking that your hotel does an early breakfast, by investing some time and effort in preparation, you'll save yourself stress and maximise your chances of putting in a good performance.

Appendix 1:
URINE COLOUR CHART

Urine colour charts are simple tools to help you to assess hydration level. You should aim to have urine in the 1–3 bands. If your urine is darker (4–8), this would suggest you need to drink more fluid.

Be aware that some multivitamin supplements can affect the colour of your urine, reducing the validity of this chart. In this case you should consider other methods of monitoring hydration such as weight as described in Chapter 3 (see page 45).

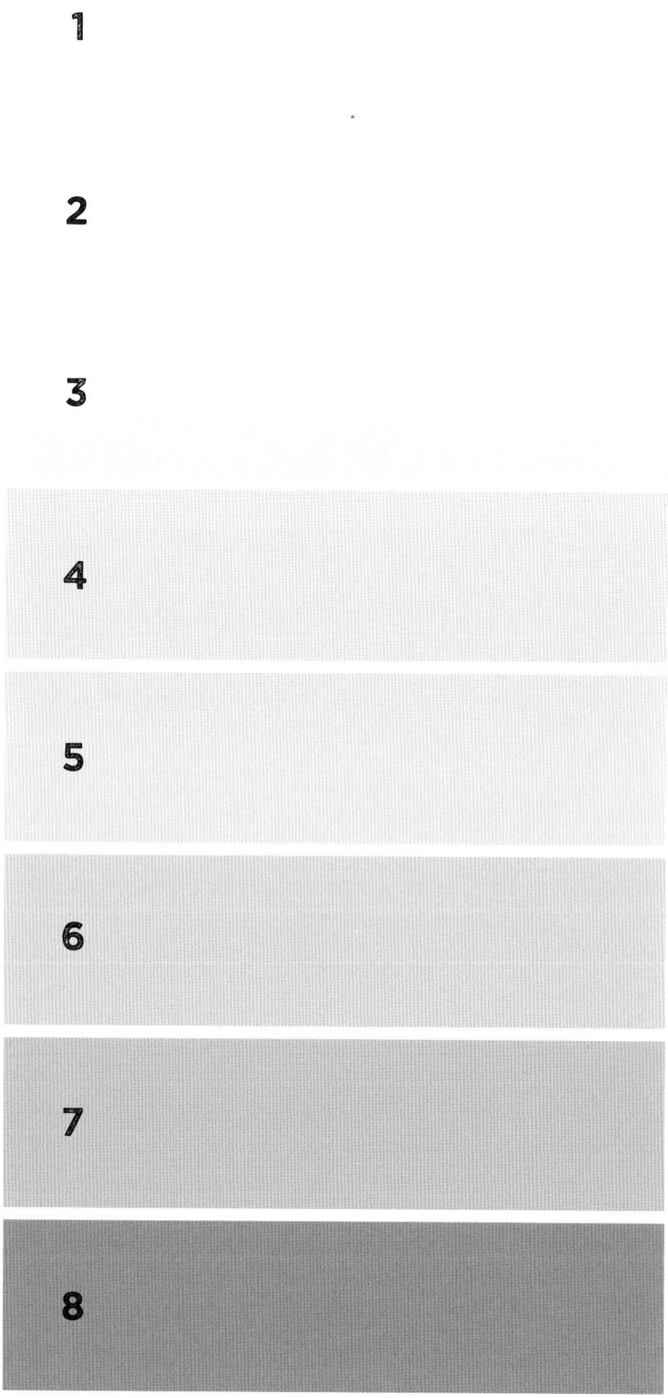

1

2

3

4

5

6

7

8

Appendix 2: CARBOHYDRATE EXCHANGE LIST READY RECKONER

FOOD PORTIONS CONTAINING 50g OF CARBOHYDRATE				
Food	Approximate weight		Common measure	GI (Pure glucose = 100)
	Grams	Oz		
Breakfast cereals				
Porridge (made with water and milk)	500	20	1 large bowl	50
Weetabix	75	3	3–4 biscuits	75
Shredded Wheat	75	3	3 biscuits	70
Shreddies	75	3	1 large bowl	65
Bran Flakes	75	3	1 large bowl	70
Cornflakes	50	2	1 large bowl	80
Muesli	75	3	1 medium bowl	50
All-Bran	50	2	1 large bowl	60
Cereals and grains				
Quinoa	80 (raw)	3	2 tbsp	35
Pasta: white or wholewheat (cooked)	225	9	8 tbsp	40
Rice: white (cooked)	175	7	4 tbsp	65
Rice: basmati (cooked)	175	7	4 tbsp	50
Tinned spaghetti in tomato sauce	400	16	1 large can	70
Tinned ravioli	500	20	1 large can	65
Pulses				
Baked beans	325	13	7 tbsp	55
Sweetcorn/corn	300	12	10 tbsp	60
Red kidney beans	300	12	10 tbsp	50
Chickpeas	275	11	10 tbsp	40

FOOD PORTIONS CONTAINING 50g OF CARBOHYDRATE

Food	Approximate weight		Common measure	GI (Pure glucose = 100)
	Grams	Oz		
Potatoes				
Boiled	300	12	5 egg size	60
Jacket/skin	175	7	1 medium	50
Sweet potato	175	7	1 medium	40
Mashed	325	13	5 scoops	70
Chips/fries	175	7	¾ chip shop portion	75
Roast	200	8	4 small	75
Crisps	100	4	4 packets	55
Low-fat crisps	75	3	3 packets	50
Bakery products				
White bread	100	4	3–4 slices	70
Wholemeal bread	125	5	3–4 slices	60
Rolls	100	4	2	70
Pitta bread	100	4	1 large	60
Naan bread	100	4	2 mini	50
Rye bread (pumpernickel)	100	4	3 large slices	50
Tortilla wraps	100	4	1 ½ medium slices	65
Crumpets	125	5	3	69
Currant buns/teacakes	100	4	1–2	90
Fruit scones	100	4	2	50
Malt loaf	100	4	2–3 slices	72
Bagels	75	3	1	70
Jam tarts	75	3	3	70
Swiss roll	100	4	3 slices	70
Cereal bars and desserts				
Jordans Fruesli (Fruit & Nut)	80	3	2 ½ bars	75
Jordans Original Crunchy	80	3	2 ½ bars	75
Tracker (Nut)	80	3	3 bars	75
Nutrigrain Bars	70	3	2 bars	65
Jelly	70	3	½ packet	85

FOOD PORTIONS CONTAINING 50g OF CARBOHYDRATE

Food	Approximate weight		Common measure	GI (Pure glucose = 100)
	Grams	Oz		
Fruits				
Apples	425	17	4 medium	40
Oranges	625	25	4 medium	40
Pears	525	21	3 medium	40
Bananas	225	9	2 large	55
Dried apricots	150	6	20	30
Dates (dried)	100	4	7	100
Figs (dried)	100	4	5	60
Raisins	75	3	3 tbsp	65
Grapes	325	13	60	50
Peaches in juice	500	20	1 large can	50
Pineapple in juice	400	16	1 large can	60
Apricots in juice	400	16	1 ½ large cans	65
Biscuits				
Plain digestive	75	3	5	60
Ginger nuts	75	3	7	70
Fig rolls	125	5	4–5	65
Jaffa Cake	75	3	6	70
Oatcakes	75	3	6	57
Crispbread, such as Ryvita	75	3	9	65
Crackers	75	3	10	65
Rice cakes	75	3	10	70
Dairy foods				
Rice pudding (low-fat)	325	13	1 can	60
Ice cream	225	9	4 scoops	50
Custard (low-fat)	425	17	1 can	40
Milk – whole, semi or skimmed	11	40	2 pints	40

FOOD PORTIONS CONTAINING 50g OF CARBOHYDRATE

Food	Approximate weight		Common measure	GI (Pure glucose = 100)
	Grams	Oz		
Confectionery				
Milk or plain chocolate	75	3	1 ½ 50g bars	50
KitKat	75	3	8 fingers	55
Milky Way	75	3	1 ½ bars	55
Mars	75	3	1 bar	70
Bounty	100	4	1 ½ bars	60
Snickers	100	4	1 ½ bars	60
Jelly Babies	75	3	1 medium packet	80
Liquorice Allsorts	75	3	1 medium bag	70
Fruit Pastilles	75	3	2 tubes	70
Sugar/preserves				
White or brown sugar	50	2	12 level tsp	95
Jam	75	3	9 level tsp	60
Honey	75	3	9 level tsp	50
Syrup	75	3	9 level tsp	75
Drinks				
Fruit juice	550	22	1 pint	50
Ribena (diluted)	400	16	2 glasses	60
Cola	500	20	1 ½ cans	60
Lemonade	800	32	2 ½ cans	60
Lucozade (original)	250	10	1 glass	95
Isotonic sports drink	600	24	2 bottles	75

Sources: *adapted from McCance R.A., Widdowson, E.M. (1991) The Composition of Foods*. London: Royal Society of Chemistry Publishing. Crawley, H. (1988). *Food Portion Sizes*, 2nd ed. London: HMSO. www.glycemicindex.com, University of Sydney.

Appendix 3: READY RECKONER OF PROTEIN FOODS

Food portions containing approximately 20 g of animal protein

Animal source	Approximate weight		Handy measure
Beef, lamb, pork	75 g	3 oz	2 medium slices
Turkey, chicken	75 g	3 oz	1 small breast
Liver	100 g	4 oz	2 tbsp
Grilled fish	100 g	4 oz	1 small fillet
Fish fingers	100 g	4 oz	6 fishfingers
Salmon/tuna	100 g	4 oz	1 small tin
Sardines	100 g	4 oz	1 small tin
Prawns (shrimps)	100 g	4 oz	2 tbsp
Cockles	200 g	8 oz	4 tbsp
Eggs	–	–	3 medium
Cheddar cheese	75 g	3 oz	2 matchbox size pieces
Edam cheese	150 g	6 oz	2 matchbox size pieces
Cottage cheese	150 g	6 oz	4 tbsp
Milk – skimmed/semi-skimmed	600 ml	24 fl oz	1 pint
Low-fat yoghurt	400 ml	16 fl oz	3 cartons

Food portions containing approximately 10 g of vegetable protein.

Vegetable source	Approximate weight		Handy measure
Nuts (e.g. peanuts, cashews)	50 g	2 oz	1 medium packet
Seeds (e.g. sunflower, sesame)	50 g	2 oz	4 tbsp
Baked beans	200 g	8 oz	4 tbsp
Kidney beans/split peas (cooked)	150 g	6 oz	5 tbsp
Lentils (cooked)	150 g	6 oz	5 tbsp
Tofu (soya bean curd)	125 g	5 oz	½ packet
Soya milk	350 ml	14 fl oz	approx. ⅔ pint
Houmous	125 g	5 oz	3 tbsp
Peanut butter	50 g	2 oz	Thickly spread on 2 slices of bread
Bread	125 g	5 oz	4 large slices
Pasta/noodles	250 g	10oz	8 tbsp – cooked
Plain rice (cooked)	450 g	18 oz	12 tbsp – cooked
Cornflakes	100 g	4 oz	2 large bowls
Rice Krispies	150 g	6 oz	3 large bowls
Weetabix	100 g	4 oz	5 Weetabix
Digestive biscuits	100 g	4 oz	7 biscuits
Semi sweet biscuits	150 g	6 oz	6–8 biscuits

Sources: *adapted from McCance R. A., Widdowson, E. M. (1991) The Composition of Foods.* London: Royal Society of Chemistry Publishing.
Crawley, H. (1988). *Food Portion Sizes*, 2nd ed. London: HMSO.

Appendix 4: CONVERSION CHART FOR COMMON MEASUREMENTS

U.S.	Metric
1 teaspoon	5 milliliters
1 tablespoon (3 teaspoons)	15 milliliters
1 fluid ounce (2 tablespoons)	30 milliliters
¼ cup	60 milliliters
⅓ cup	80 milliliters
½ cup	120 milliliters
1 cup	240 milliliters
1 pint (2 cups)	480 milliliters
1 quart (4 cups; 32 ounces)	960 milliliters
1 gallon (4 quarts)	3.84 liters
1 ounce (by weight)	28 grams
1 pound	454 grams
2.2 pounds	1 kilogram

OVEN TEMPERATURES

°F	Gas mark	°C
250	½	120
275	1	140
300	2	150
325	3	165
350	4	180
375	5	190
400	6	200
425	7	220
450	8	230
475	9	240
500	10	260

ACKNOWLEDGMENTS

I would like to take this opportunity to thank a few people, who, without their help and support, this book would never have been possible. Firstly I have to thank my mother, not only because her terrible cooking made me want to be better, but because from her I learned the love of sport and how hard work results in reward. I must also thank all of the athletes that I worked with over the years; not only stars such as Mark Cavendish, Sir Bradley Wiggins, Sir Chris Hoy, Chris Froome and Victoria Pentleton, but also all the other athletes who work just as hard but do not necessarily receive the same recognition.

I would like to pay a special thanks to Sir Dave Brailsford, without whom the doors would never have been opened for the likes of me to walk through. Finally my biggest thanks goes to my wife Julie, who makes everything possible for me.

Photo Credits

Diagrams on page 26 by Dave Saunders © Bloomsbury Publishing

Photos on pages 72–73, 88, 90, 113, 114, 137, 138, 159, 160, 186, 197, 198 by Adrian Lawrence Photography © Bloomsbury Publishing

Photos on pages 10, 14, 19, 24, 32, 35, 40, 44, 48, 51, 58, 64, 74, 77, 78, 118, 123, 126, 132, 144, 163, 174, 188, 203, 208, 213, 217, 220, 224 © Getty Images

Photos on pages 62–63, 93, 99 © Presse Sport/Offside

INDEX

A

acidity, stomach 27, 29–30, 37
alcohol 17, 37, 45, 63, 130, 151
alkaline levels, intestine 27, 29, 37, 173
amino acids 13, 36, 47, 49, 122, 124, 154, 176–7, 179, 190–1
antibiotics 32, 36, 172
antioxidants 166–7, 173
Armitstead, Lizzie 190
author's background 7–9

B

B vitamins 60, 192
bacteria, gut 27–8, 31, 34, 36, 37, 171–2, 204
bananas 46, 49, 61, 80, 163
beetroot juice 178, 186
beta-alanine 176–7, 192
blood sugar levels 59, 60, 61, 110
body composition 141–3, 145, 157
bone health 149–50, 207
bonking 68, 110, 111
bowel movements 28, 66
branch chain amino acids (BCAAs) 47, 49, 155–6, 179
bread 13, 33, 79, 200, 204
breakfasts
    day before an event 60–1
    eggs 75–6, 78, 80
    on event day 75–86
    gut rehab 33–4
    how much to eat 80
    hydration 79–80
    low-residue 38
    porridge 60, 75–7, 80, 87, 90–1, 204
    recipes 87–91
    rice pudding 81
    when to eat 80, 84
    see also timelines, nutritional
British Cycling 6, 8, 9, 95, 129, 183
buffers 175–8
Burton, Beryl 209

C

caffeine 37, 61, 79–80, 130, 173–4
calcium 53, 150, 205, 207, 210
calorie calculations 147–9, 157
camomile tea and honey 62–3, 75
Caprese salad 160
carbohydrate-fasted rides 15, 49, 106–8, 120, 223
carbohydrates 9, 11, 12–13, 34, 49, 204
    breakfast on event day 80, 81
    day before an event 59, 61–2
    Glycemic Index 60
    during heavy training 149, 209
    junior riders 210
    metabolic recovery 120–2
    pasta loading 59, 68, 200
    ready reckoner 229–32
    sports drinks 45, 46–7, 49, 50, 53, 56–7, 79
    weight loss 152
    see also gluten-free diets; nutrition
carnosine 176–7
casein proteins 62, 124, 156
chain gang nutrition, evening 101–2
chewing your food 26
chicken/poultry 33, 34, 61, 177
    with rice and quinoa 69
    turkey breast steak with sweet potato wedges and spinach 70
    turkey burgers 158
    turkey power soup 185
chocolate, seed, nut and berry porridge topping 91
cholesterol in eggs 78
Clancy, Ed 154
coeliac disease 201, 202
coffee and tea 37, 45, 79–80, 175, 191
colas 30, 37, 129
colon/large intestine 27–8, 29
colostrum 36, 172
commutes, nutrition for working day 223–4
compression clothing 65–6, 131
Cook, Nicole 209
cottage cheese 156

cramps 53, 55
creatine 155, 176, 177–8, 192
Cummings, Steve 183
cyclocross race, nutrition for mid-morning 221–2

D

D, vitamin 20, 23, 150, 170
dairy foods 16, 30, 33, 122, 124, 190, 192
dairy-free diets 204–5, 206, 211
dehydration 42, 43, 146
    see also hydration
diaries, keeping food 151–2
diets, fad 152–3, 157, 211
digestive system 26–9, 200, 205
    see also gut health
Dombrowski, Joe 155–6
doping see drugs
drinks see alcohol; energy drinks; hydration; recovery drinks; sports drinks; water
drugs/drug tests 8, 180–1, 182–3

E

early-morning time trial 218–20
eating on the bike 6–7, 15, 34
    evening chain gang 101–2
    female riders 207
    gluten free 204
    junior riders 210
    short turbo session 106
    sportives 99–101
    steady-paced endurance rides 97–9
    structured intervals in training 103, 106
    wrapping your food 117
    see also nutrition
eggs 33, 75–6, 80, 122, 190
eicosapentaenoic acid (EPA) 127, 128, 170–1, 182–3, 184
electrolytes 41, 46–7, 49, 50, 53, 55
endurance rides, nutrition for steady-paced 97–9
energised greens 34, 172–3

energy balance estimate 146–9
energy balls recipe 115
energy bars and drinks 49, 81, 84, 163, 184, 204
enzymes 15, 26, 27, 200
ergogenic aids 163, 164, 173–9
Erythropoietin (EPO) 182
essential amino acids 13, 122
essential fatty acids 8, 16, 192–3
    see also omega-3 fatty acids
evening crit nutrition 215–18
evening track league nutrition 218
evolution, human 142, 145

F

faecal mass 28, 31, 34, 37
fat, body 12, 16, 59, 141–3, 145
fats 8, 11, 16–17, 125–6, 149, 152, 207
feed stations 47, 101, 111, 213
female riders 143, 167, 207, 209, 211
fermented foods 34, 36, 172
fibre 13, 27–8, 31, 37, 66, 173, 204
fish and seafood 33, 36, 61, 122, 127, 171
fish oil 8, 16, 156, 207
five-bean chilli recipe 196
flaxseeds 16, 171, 193, 198
food intolerances 30, 201–2, 204–6
food processor/juicers 22
free radicals 166
Froome, Chris 6, 7, 54, 110
fructose 12, 47, 49, 62–3, 96
fruit 13, 31, 61, 66, 166–7, 204
    juices 45, 96, 125
Functional Threshold Heart Rate (FTHR) 95
Functional Threshold Power (FRP) 95, 153

G

gastrointestinal issues 29, 32, 33, 49, 66, 200–2
gels 96, 110, 163, 184, 204
Giro d'Italia Grand Tour 8, 156, 226
glow nutrients (micronutrients) 17–18, 23, 59, 66, 173, 210
glucosamine 166
glucose 12, 47, 96, 110, 204

glutamine 36, 173
gluten 30, 33, 200
gluten-free diets 200–4, 206, 211
Glycemic Index 60, 75–6, 121–2
glycogen 12, 15, 16, 43, 59, 68, 75, 108, 110, 120–2
go nutrients (macronutrients) 11–13, 15–17, 23, 59, 163, 184
grains 33, 190, 200, 204
Grand Tours
    energy balance 147
    Giro d'Italia 8, 156, 226
    hydration 21, 54
    nutrition 8, 13, 15, 25, 121, 124
    Old School vs Modern diet 21
    recovery 119, 121, 129, 130, 131
    substituting EPO for EPA 182–3
    Tour de France 22, 110, 129
    Tour of California 65
    travelling 65
Great Britain Cycling Team 6, 183
gut flora *see* bacteria, gut
gut health 9, 13, 25, 39, 171–3
    alkalinity and acidity 27, 29–30, 37
    easily-digestible diet 34, 36
    gut rehab plan 33–4, 173, 202
    low-residue diets 37–8
    stressors 28–31, 39
gym work 153, 154, 155, 157, 209

H

heart rate monitors 93, 147, 213
herbal teas 52, 61
honey 52, 62–3
hormones 15, 149, 207
hydration 41–3
    breakfast on event day 79–80
    can you drink too much? 52
    in the cold 50, 52
    cramps 53, 55
    Grand Tours 21, 54
    how much to drink on the bike 45–6
    off the bike 43, 45
    recovery 55, 124
    timing drinking on the bike 46
    what to drink on the bike 46–7, 49–50
hygiene 29
hypertonic solutions 50

hyponatremia 52
hypotonic solutions 50

I

ice baths 132–3
illness 152, 157
immune system 15, 25, 26, 29, 34, 170, 173, 201
injuries 152, 157, 166
intensity, monitoring riding 93–5, 111, 213
iron 20, 23, 167–9, 183, 191, 201, 207
isotonic solutions 45, 50

J

James, Becky 209
jet lag 65
juicers 22
juices, fruit 45, 96, 125
juices, vegetable 34, 37, 45, 66, 125, 167, 178, 186–7, 204
junior riders 210, 211

K

Kappes, Anthony 202
kefir 36, 172
ketones 145–6, 181
kitchen essentials 22

L

l-carnitine 179
lactate and acid 175–6
lactose 30, 33, 36
    dairy-free diets 204–5, 206
leaky gut 31, 34
leg elevation 130–1
legumes 53, 190, 205
leucine 155–6, 179
London 2012 Olympic Games 96, 129
low-residue diets 37–8, 66

M

mackerel and tomato salad 139
MacLean, Craig 202
magnesium supplements 53
maltodextrin 12, 47, 49, 96, 204

massage 131
measuring riding intensity 93–5, 111
meat 13, 16, 33, 37, 61, 122, 192
medications, pain 133
menstruation 167, 207
metabolic recovery 119, 120–1, 134
Milan–San Remo race 80
milk, cow's 30, 33, 36, 124, 156, 163, 204–5
milk substitutes 33, 192
minerals 18, 20, 23, 167–9
    see also iron; supplements, dietary
Montmorency cherry juice 167
multivitamins and multi-minerals 20, 23, 167–70, 183
    see also supplements, dietary
muscle 15, 53
    body composition 141–2
    female riders 207, 209
    gaining 153–6
    glycogen 43, 59, 108, 110, 120–2
    l-carnitine supplements 179
    losing muscle mass 142, 145–6, 152–3, 209
    muscular recovery 119, 122, 124, 209

N

nerves, event 66
nitrates 178
nutrition
    10-mile time trial 215–18
    breakfast on event day 75–91
    day before and event 59, 60–3, 68, 70–1
    early-morning time trials 218–20
    evening chain gang 101–2
    evening crit 215–18
    evening track league 218
    how the pros fuel their rides 67–8, 85, 108–9
    intensity of riding 93–5, 213
    long training rides 213–15
    mid-morning cyclocross race 221–2
    short turbo sessions 106
    sportives 99–101, 213–15
    steady-paced endurance rides 97–9
    structured intervals in training 103, 106

whilst travelling to an event 63, 65, 66, 69
    working day with commutes 223–4
    see also eating on the bike; gut health; hydration; recovery
nuts 53, 61, 190

O

oats, porridge see porridge oats
Olympic Games, Atlanta 1996 8
Olympic Games, London 2012 96, 129
Olympic Games, Rio 2016 142
Olympic Games, Sydney 2000 202
omega-3s fatty acids 16, 36, 125–8, 156, 170–1, 182, 192–3, 207
omega-6 170–1, 193
omelettes 15, 61, 75, 78, 80, 88
osmolarity 49–50
osmotic pressure 47

P

painkillers 133
panini recipe, traditional 116
Paralympics London 2012
Paris–Roubaix, fuelling the 67–8, 85
pasta 13, 33, 59, 68, 200, 204
Pendleton, Victoria 209
pH levels, gut 27, 29–30, 37, 49
pickles 36, 172
pistachio pâté with sweet potato wedges and wilted spinach 71
plant-based protein sources 190–1, 205, 234
plant cellulose 13
plant foods see fruit; grains; nuts and seeds; porridge oats; vegetables
porridge oats 13, 60, 75–7, 80, 87, 90–1, 204
Porte, Riche 110
power meters 9, 93–5, 147, 213
prebiotics 27, 31, 37, 171, 204
probiotics 34, 36, 171–2
processed weight-loss food 152–3, 157
protein 8, 11, 13, 15, 129, 145, 233–4
    dairy-free diets 205
    day before an event 59, 61, 62
    female riders 207, 209

importance of 129, 149, 152, 154
muscular recovery 122, 124, 209
plant-based sources 190–1, 205, 234
powders/supplements 34, 124, 150, 164–5
ready reckoner 233–4
recovery and sports drinks 47, 49, 156, 163, 191
vegans and vegetarians 190–1
    see also eggs; fish; gluten; meat; nutrition; poultry
psychological recovery 119

Q

quinoa 62, 204
    and coconut milk porridge 90

R

recovery 55, 119
    eating on rest days 128
    foods to boost 125–8
    leg elevation 130–1
    light riding 131–2
    maximising your 130–3
    metabolic 119, 120–1, 134
    muscular 119, 122, 124, 134
    psychological 119
    recipes 135–9
recovery drinks 46, 102, 106, 108, 119, 121, 124–5, 135, 156, 163, 191
rest days, eating on 128
rice 34, 61–2, 78
rice cake recipe 112
rice cakes 7, 9, 31, 34, 49, 81, 84, 117, 204
rice cookers 22
rice pudding 81
Rowsell Shand, Joanna 209

S

salads 34, 61, 62, 173
    Caprese 160
    dressings 191
    mackerel and tomato 139
saturated fats 16–17
Sciandri, Max 9
seeds 16, 36, 53, 61, 77, 78, 171,

190
skin-fold assessments 143, 145, 146, 148, 157
sleep 61, 63, 75, 81, 130
slow cookers 22
    five-bean chilli 196
    recovery stew 136
small intestines 27, 28, 33, 37, 200
smoothies
    soya, chia and flaxseed 198
    super-green 187
sodium bicarbonate 176–7
soft drinks/sodas 37, 45, 129
soup, turkey power 185
soya based foods 191, 192
soya, chia and flaxseed smoothies 198
spiced food 62, 66
sportives, fuelling 99–101, 213–15
sports drinks 25, 29–30, 37, 41, 45, 47, 49–50, 53, 79
    homemade sports drinks 56–7
Spring Classics 54, 67
starches 12, 13
stew recipe, recovery 136
Storey, Dame Sarah 209
stretching 53, 130
sugars see fructose; glucose
super-green smoothie 187
supplements, dietary 36, 39, 53, 155–6, 163–4, 184
    eicosapentaenoic acid (EPA) 127, 128, 170–1, 182–3, 184
    ergogenic supplements 173–9
    health and well-being supplements 165–7
    ketones 145–6, 181
    multivitamins and multi-minerals 20, 23, 167–70, 183, 192
    omega-3 oils 36, 170–1, 207
    probiotics and prebiotics 171–2
    protein powders 34, 124, 150, 164–5, 191
    quality assurance 180–1
sweat tests 45, 55
sweating 42, 43
sweet potatoes 61

T

tea and coffee see coffee and tea; herbal teas
Team Sky 6, 8–9, 15, 22, 76, 121, 129, 130, 183, 226
teenage riders 210, 211
testosterone 78
time trials, nutrition for 10-mile 215–18
timelines, nutritional
    10-mile time trial 215–18
    early-morning time trial 218–20
    evening crit 215–18
    evening track league 218
    long training rides 213–15
    mid-morning cyclocross race 221–2
    planning your own 227
    sportives 213–15
    working day with commutes 223–4
Tour de France 22, 110, 129
Tour of California 65
training and gut health 29
trans fats 16, 17
'transporters' 120
travelling to events 63, 65–6, 68
Trott, Laura 209
turbo sessions, nutrition for short 106
turkey breast steak with sweet potato wedges and wilted spinach 70
turkey burgers 158
turkey power soup 185

U

unsaturated fats 16, 17
urine colour charts 43, 45, 55, 228

V

vegan protein bars 199
vegetable oils 170–1, 193
vegetables 13, 31, 53, 61, 62, 66, 122, 166–7, 172–3, 191, 204, 210
    juices 34, 37, 45, 66, 125, 167, 178, 186–7, 204
vegetarians and vegans 13, 36, 122, 189–93, 206, 211
Very Berry Protein Fluff 161
villi 27, 28, 29, 31, 34, 36, 171, 201
vinegars 191
vitamins 18, 20, 23, 150, 167, 170, 192
    see also supplements, dietary

W

water 21, 25, 27, 34, 41, 45, 46, 61
    see also drinks; hydration
weather conditions 50, 52, 54
weight management 8, 9, 15, 42, 43, 45, 55, 141
    body composition 141–3, 145, 157
    energy balance 146–9
    fad diets and weight-loss foods 152–3
    gaining muscle/lean tissue 153–5, 209
    gym work 153, 154, 155, 157, 209
    during heavy training 149–50, 157, 207
    illness and injury 152, 157
    keeping food diaries 151–2
    losing muscle/lean tissue 142, 145–6, 152–3
    skin-fold assessments 143, 145, 146, 148, 157
wheat 30, 33, 200–2, 204
whey protein 108, 124, 179, 191, 205
Wiggins, Sir Bradley 6, 7, 8, 9, 15, 31, 54, 65, 129, 142, 182–3, 226
World Anti-Doping Agency (WADA) 180, 181
wrapping your food 117

Y

Yates, Sean 9, 16
yeast extract 192
yoghurt 33, 34, 36, 61, 62, 156

Z

Zabriskie, David 190